Sizzle & Smoke

THE ULTIMATE GUIDE TO GRILLING FOR DIABETES, PREDIABETES, AND HEART HEALTH

Chef Steven Petusevsky

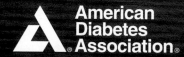

American Diabetes Association.

Director, Book Publishing, Abe Ogden; Managing Editor, Greg Guthrie; Acquisitions Editor, Victor Van Beuren; Editor, Rebekah Renshaw; Production Manager, Melissa Sprott; Composition and Cover Design, pixiedesign, llc; Photographer, Renee Comet; Printer, RR Donnelley.

Printed in the United States of America
1 3 5 7 9 10 8 6 4 2

The suggestions and information contained in this publication are generally consistent with the Clinical Practice Recommendations and other policies of the American Diabetes Association, but they do not represent the policy or position of the Association or any of its boards or committees. Reasonable steps have been taken to ensure the accuracy of the information presented. However, the American Diabetes Association cannot ensure the safety or efficacy of any product or service described in this publication. Individuals are advised to consult a physician or other appropriate health care professional before undertaking any diet or exercise program or taking any medication referred to in this publication. Professionals must use and apply their own professional judgment, experience, and training and should not rely solely on the information contained in this publication before prescribing any diet, exercise, or medication. The American Diabetes Association—its officers, directors, employees, volunteers, and members—assumes no responsibility or liability for personal orother injury, loss, or damage that may result from the suggestions or information in this publication.

⊚ The paper in this publication meets the requirements of the ANSI Standard Z39.48-1992 (permanence of paper).

ADA titles may be purchased for business or promotional use or for special sales. To purchase more than 50 copies of this book at a discount, or for custom editions of this book with your logo, contact the American Diabetes Association at the address below, at booksales@diabetes.org, or by calling 703-299-2046.

American Diabetes Association
1701 North Beauregard Street
Alexandria, Virginia 22311

DOI: 10.2337/9781580405300

Library of Congress Cataloging-in-Publication Data

Petusevsky, Steve.
  Sizzle and smoke / Steven Petusevsky.
     page cm
Includes bibliographical references and index.
  ISBN 978-1-58040-530-0 (alk. paper)
  1. Diet therapy. 2. Barbecuing. 3. Diabetes--Diet therapy--Recipes. 4. Heart--Diseases--Diet therapy--Recipes. I. American Diabetes Association. II. Title.
  RC684.D5P48 2014
  641.5'6314--dc23
                      2013044949

ACKNOWLEDGMENTS

This is the part of the book that produces post production depression for me. It's a weird dichotomy of relief and sadness. Writing is often a lonely process and forces me to live inside only my own mind for long periods of time. Sometimes this can be quite uncomfortable. Creating a book is a team effort in spite of the solitude involved and I often fear I will forget to thank people that helped these pages come to life.

First and foremost, I want to thank Abe Ogden and Rebekah Renshaw at the American Diabetes Association for believing in me and for the opportunity to write this book and hopefully reach so many people who will benefit from these pages. Thanks to Renee Comet of Renee Comet Photography and food stylist Lisa Cherkasky for their always brilliant photographs. My hope is to positively affect many readers and perhaps inspire them to begin new traditions with their families and friends. I want them to know creative healthful food is simple, beautiful, and delicious, especially on the grill!

I want to thank Lori, my fiancée for her unending support, encouragement and true acts of love. She is my soul mate and a great lover of my food, which she never fails to communicate to me, especially when I need to hear it the most. Ironically she is a vegetarian and although many of the recipes in this book are vegetarian, many others are not. Gleefully she watched as my brothers, their wives, and friends ate copious amounts of meat and smiled through it! I also want to thank and express appreciation and much love to my family: my dad Lenny who eats anything I put down in front of him. My brothers: Mitchell and Howie and their wives Wendy and Roberta, for hosting many grill parties. My kids: Sabrina and Jared have been my recipe test dummies for over 20 years now, and continue to give me immeasurable joy when I cook for them. It is equally as wonderful to have 3 step daughters who love their grilled food: Dana, Arianne, and Avital, are always honest in sharing their food thoughts.

My agent and friend for many years, Beth Shepard has always been there for me, not only to make this book a reality, but to bounce around any thoughts both food and life related. She always sorts through these inner musings in the most logical manner.

I consider myself a lucky man with so many people around me that I love and respect who inspire my global travels and unending quest for that elusive recipe, authentic cooking method, or incredible food photo that I just have to take.

I want to give thanks to my mother, Claire who was my food muse and will always be in my mind and heart. She inspired my life of food and my continuous culinary journey. She was an amazing cook even though I was 14 when I first realized fish wasn't necessarily shaped like a brick and lived in the freezer. I often ask myself, "How would mom cook this?" To my dad, Lenny, who recently passed, I'm sure my mom and dad will be reading this next book together.

Enjoy these favorite recipes, share them with loved ones, eat responsibly and always tell ones close to you how much you love them.

It's time now to fire up the grill!

Chef Steve

Table of Contents

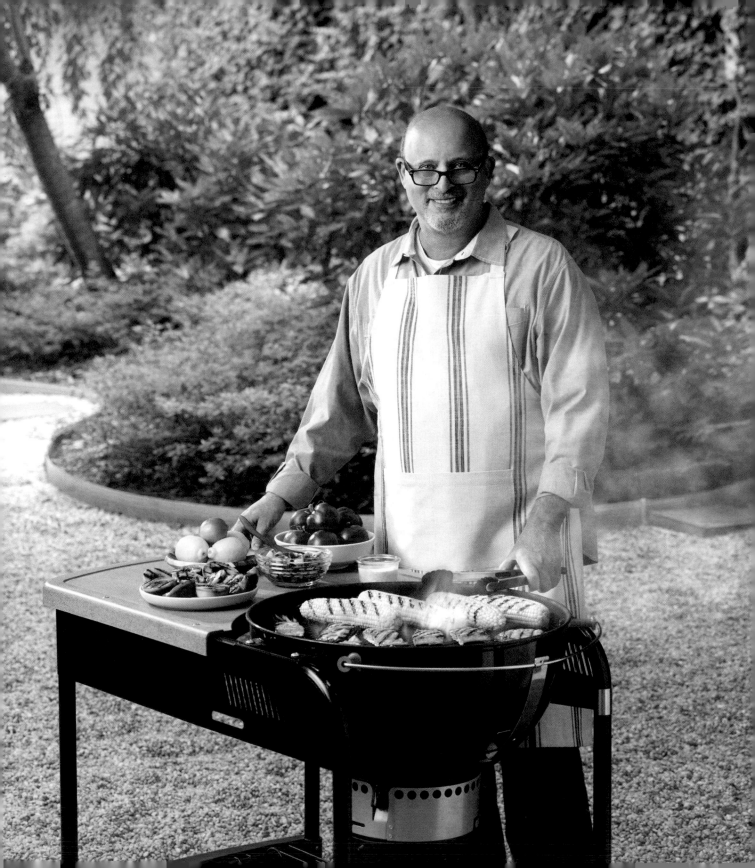

INTRODUCTION

You'll notice from the recipe titles, chapter offerings, and stunning photos that, although this book is about the art of grilling, it goes far beyond the typical grill book.

All of the recipes have been carefully designed to be nutritionally appropriate for those with diabetes, prediabetes, and for optimal heart health. The recipes are easy to follow, contain ingredients that are readily available, and are unique and creative. Many of the recipes are influenced by my personal travels and observations of other cultures. The flavors are bold with a minimum amount of fuss and kitchen toil. Plus, there are a host of recipes that accompany the grilled offerings that can be prepared in the kitchen or even the day before you plan on firing up the grill.

The Rub, Soak, and Savor chapter includes incredible marinades and simple ways to impart flavor to any grilled item, whether it is a meat, or plant-based protein. I use many of these flavoring recipes not only for home use, but when I am in the professional kitchen as well. One of my current personal favorites is Dukkah, a spice sprinkle I've been using like magic fairy dust on everything from grilled asparagus to pan-sautéed green tomatoes.

The chef in me knows that most grilled foods need a little salsa, sauce, or simple chutney to spoon over the top to highlight and kick up the flavor. The recipes you'll find in the Over the Top chapter give you some unforgettable recipes to garnish your grilled entrées.

Romesco Sauce (page 88), Satay Peanut Sauce (page 89), and Olive and Fig Tapenade (page 93) are just a few of the delightful sauces that are made to accompany your favorite grilled item.

Side dishes are often the highlight of my meal. I wanted to share with you some of my favorite items that pair with grilled foods. Combining several vegetarian recipes makes for the perfect dinner for your family and guests even if they are not practicing vegetarians. The Center of the Plate chapter is immense and covers everything from creative vegetarian dishes to every sort of meat, seafood, and poultry.

In this book, you will find Grilled Clams with Garlic (Butter) and Lime (page 52) and Grilled Seafood and Quinoa Salad with Mango and Avocado (page 79). The Peruvian Super Chicken (page 20) is incredible, and the Bahn Mi Sandwich (page 70) will blow you away. These recipes are eclectic in spectrum, with authentic flavor. Plus, they are easy to prepare.

The Desserts chapter contains mostly fruit-based desserts. Changing with the seasons, each of the recipes is worthy of company, but can bring the entire family to the dinner table any night of the week.

To your health and a hot grill,

Steven Petusevsky

GRILLING SECRETS AND TIPS

Grilling meat over an open fire began thousands of years ago, shortly after man figured out how to make and control fire. Grilling as we know it only took off in the late 1940's and early 1950's when mass-produced barbeque grills became available and the concept really caught on. It was post–World War II and dads were home from the war, the suburbs were booming, neighborhoods were being built, and many now had a backyard with a patio or a deck. Parks were being built everywhere and interest in outdoor dining as a pastime became prevalent across America. It was time to celebrate and America's taste for grilling at home exploded and has continued ever since.

The first taste of "barbeque" came from the Spanish "baracoa" and spread to the Arawak Indians of the Caribbean. The Arawak would thread bits of meat and whole fish on skewers and grill them over open fire. I offer you this information because several of the recipes in this book were taught to me on my many trips to Jamaica where Arawak descendants were said to create the grill technique that we now know as jerk or jerk cooking. In fact the Jamaican Stuffed Fish with Ritz (page 43) is prepared today in the same manner as it was centuries ago.

Okay, history lesson is over. Let's get down to basics.

Unless you are a professional competitor or true barbecue aficionado, there are two main outdoor forms of grilling that most of us really care about: gas or charcoal grills. In the charcoal category, I also include wood, natural charcoal, or briquettes. You can have grills that offer a combination of gas ignition, which light your wood or coals as well, and that's my preferred route. I love the taste of wood, and the gas ignition makes things even easier.

If you are going the coal or wood route, you will need a fire starter box. A fire starter box is a cylindrical can with a handle in which you build or stack your coals. This allows the coals to ignite faster, as they are layered vertically.

There's one more aspect of grilling to consider— indoor grilling. Consider the actual definition of grilling first. Grilling is a form of cooking that involves dry heat applied to the surface of food, commonly from above or below. It is sometimes referred to as "barbecuing," but that word also means a specific technique and flavor profile. For our purposes, grilling remains consistent with its definition.

I love my grill pan. If you don't feel like setting up your grill outside, or live in a place that has four seasons, consider a grill pan. It's my all-time favorite kitchen tool. Mine is rectangular, has raised ridges over the bottom surface, which emulate the wires of a grill. After searing your dinner on top of the stove, most grill pans can be placed in the oven much like a gas or charcoal grill. You can make a perfect steak, chicken breast, seafood filet, or thick slice of marinated fresh tofu in a grill pan, and honestly, it's the next best thing to taking the party outside.

Go ahead and read through this book, pick out recipes that pique your interest and taste buds, fire up your charcoal or gas grill, break out your grill pan, and start grilling. You, your friends, and your family will be glad you did. I hope that these simple, globally inspired recipes will become your new grilled favorites.

MAKING SURE ALL THE ELEMENTS OF YOUR DINNER ARE DONE AT ONCE

Always make all the other components first as they will hold while your grilled food cooks. I make the side dishes, salsas or relish, salads and anything else first, often starting the day before. The grilled item goes on last and everything else should be ready to go as soon as the grill gets turned off.

GRILL HEATING METHODS

Grilling is really a craft. Whether you grill over gas, wood, charcoal, or any other fuel, it's a learned technique and is quite intuitive, even though you may go through a lot of burnt food along the way. The purpose of this little information piece is to share some solid general tips on grilling. Most backyard and balcony cooks have their own family methods and little tweaks that make them the master of their own grill.

Here are a few foundational grilling tips that you can rely on if you need to. You can, of course, use our recipes, but grill the recipes in your own individual way. There are really two major methods for grilling your favorite recipes: direct and indirect heat method.

DIRECT HEAT METHOD

Wood, charcoal, or gas are the most common heating methods for grilling. The important thing here is searing or sealing the outside of your steak, chop, rib, chicken breast, vegetable, or seafood ingredient. Searing produces that amazing caramelized crust full of flavor and appeal. It is the best method for ingredients that take less than 15–20 minutes to cook. Think steaks, chops, burgers, fish filets, tofu, vegetable steaks, chicken breasts, and shellfish. Direct heat is how you make those cool crosshatch marks.

CHARCOAL OR WOOD | Build your fire. After it is ready and the coals are glowing, spread them out evenly. Put your food on the grill, close the cover, and turn the items after about 5 minutes in the opposite direction to mark the surface. Flip the food over after about 10 minutes on the grill and repeat the process. Keep your grill closed the whole time and don't make the common mistake of constantly turning your dinner, as it will not cook evenly.

GAS GRILL | Turn the burners up high. Get the grill grate really hot, lightly oil, and place your items directly on the grill. Proceed the same way, marking your ingredients with a crosshatch, close the grill, and turn it over halfway through. Test for doneness before removing from grill.

INDIRECT HEAT METHOD

This is sort of like using your grill as an oven or a convection oven. The heat from the grill rises, radiates off the inside cover and sides of grill, and cooks your ingredient through from all sides. This method is usually employed for larger cuts of meat like a turkey breast, whole chicken, ribs, roast, or whole filet mignon.

CHARCOAL OR WOOD | First put a disposable aluminum pan in the center of your grill bottom. Build your fire on one side of the grill. When coals are hot, rearrange them in an even layer around the pan in the center. Fill the small disposable aluminum pan in the center with water. This pan will disperse heat more evenly and add moisture to larger cuts of meat and poultry. It will also prevent fat from flaring up and burning. When larger cuts are cooked this way, you only have to turn them occasionally. Always cook with the lid closed.

GRILL TOOLS AND TIPS

Often I go to friends' homes and family events and people love to show me their latest gadgets. I am so amused by all the things, which someone invents, which I never needed through an entire career of cooking! Here's what my grill arsenal looks like:

- CHIMNEY STARTER | This allows you to start your fire efficiently without even using a fuel starter. You can get these everywhere.

- LONG-HANDLED TONGS | Go for the longest ones available from 16–24 inches, preferably with an insulated handle.

- LONG-HANDLED BASTING BRUSH | I love to lather on that marinade or sauce, and a long brush will save you all of those embarrassing burns and that seared arm hair.

- LONG-HANDLED TURNER OR SPATULA | for flipping burgers, tofu slabs, vegetables, etc.

- PERFORATED GRILL TRAY | for vegetables and fish filets. These make it easy to cook delicate items evenly and remove them from the grill without breaking them up.

- SPRAY BOTTLE | filled with water to cool hot spots on your grill and slow the cooking process in very hot areas of the grill.

- LONG-HANDLED WIRE BRUSH | for grill cleaning. I sometimes use the fibrous heat-resistant brushes.

- THERMOMETER

- NIGHT LIGHT | for evening grilling in the dark. Sometimes to be entertaining, I'll wear one of those mining lights that mount to a headband. You can find these inexpensively at discount stores.

- CLEAN KITCHEN TOWELS | to wipe off grill and use as a pot holder.

- CAST IRON SMOKE BOX | can hold wood chips to grill and lightly smoke your grilled items.

- SALT AND PEPPER MILLS | to season items right off the grill.

GAS GRILL | You may want to wrap your roast or meat item loosely in foil before placing on grill. Turn occasionally while basting with a sauce or marinade and keep the pan filled with water while cooking. You will want to lower the flames on each side of the metal pan to a lower setting to cook slow and evenly.

You can add a small heavy cast iron metal smoke box for wood chips, which come in all types and flavors. These are easy to use and are widely available.

WHERE THERE IS SMOKE

Using certain kinds of hardwood to flavor and smoke your foods gives them an incredible taste that's hard to beat. I find the best way to flavor even on a gas grill is to buy a cast iron smoke box. You can find these at every home improvement or grill store. Smoke boxes are used with wood chips and these come in many varieties. Apple, mesquite, hickory, cherry, and oak are my favorites, although you can now buy grapevine trimmings, which provide interesting flavor as well. Corncobs, maple wood, blackberry, and cedar are also commonly available and create delicate sweet smoke. I've recently seen old wine barrels made into chips, which I look forward to trying. If you can find pimento wood or allspice chips, which are used for making jerk chicken, there is no taste quite like it anywhere.

All of these wood chip varieties need to be soaked overnight. I keep a small bucket of them soaking next to my grill on any given day. Remember to never use wood trimmings from any building projects around the house, as they are treated with harmful chemicals.

PAIRING BEER AND WINE WITH FLAVORS OF THE GRILL

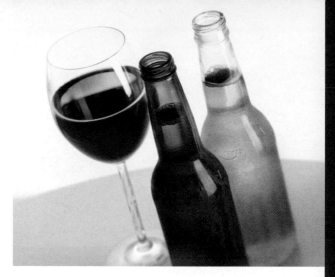

Pairing the right beer or wine with grilled foods is sort of like choosing art. In the end it all boils down to picking something you like and you think others will enjoy. Grilled foods are a little different when it comes to pairing because the strong flavors and high heat of the grill require that a strong-flavored beer or wine be served along with them.

When cooking seafood or poultry on the grill, proteins caramelize and intense flavors develop that you don't get in a sauté pan or saucepot. The same strong flavors develop around vegetables, which contain large amounts of natural sugar.

Often, I find myself pairing the ethnic background of my menu with the regions of origin for wine and beer. If I am cooking Italian, French, German, or Spanish, I'll likely select a wine from the same region.

Beers have come a long way and now make a perfect companion to grilled dishes. Microbrew beer makers are on par with serious wine makers and the selection available today makes throwing barbecues even more interesting.

Here are some of my favorite wines and beer picks to serve when grilling.

WHITE WINE

RIESLING | go for the nonsweet, not late harvest variety. My house Riesling is Bonny Doon Pacific Rim Riesling. The flavor goes with all grilled foods and it is very reasonably priced.

NEW ZEALAND SAUVIGNON BLANC | fruity, bold flavor, just the right acid tartness and reasonable in price, that's why I like these.

RED WINE

You can't go wrong with a Cabernet, Zinfandel, Pinot Noir, Tempranillo, or Malbec. Try and pair the wine with the nationality of the dish.

BEERS

WHEAT OR PILSNER BEERS | I love these effervescent, yeasty selections with lighter foods, seafood, and desserts. They go extremely well and are typically served with a slice of lemon or orange, making them a great summer pairing.

BROWN BEERS, ALES, AND AMBER BEERS | the beers pair nicely with poultry and strong seafood like swordfish or tuna steaks. You can even serve with beef, pizza, and flatbreads.

STOUTS, IMPERIAL STOUTS, AND CHOCOLATE STOUTS | these are bold and intense beers that I love. Serve these with beef, pork, lamb, and desserts. They stand up to everything but will take over if served with anything too delicate.

IPA | IPA's have an herbaceous, hoppy flavor and go well with spicy, full-bodied foods. Nothing goes better with Creole, New Orleans–inspired dishes and hot, spicy wings or Thai food.

CHAPTER 1
Rub, Soak, and Savor

Most people believe that grilling is 100% about technique; however, the true flavor comes from what you choose to rub on to the surface of the meat, fish, or poultry, or what you choose to marinate it in before you place it on the grill.

I love the eclectic nature of this chapter, because there are no culinary boundaries and the flavors come from all over the world. These recipes are favorites that I've saved through the years. The Black Coffee Mojo Marinade (page 17) comes from a family pig roast in South Florida many years ago at a time when I was surprised to see black coffee used as an ingredient. My new favorite is Dukkah Spice Sprinkle (page 12), which is my version of a Turkish spice mixture shared with me by a chef friend. I find myself sprinkling it on just about everything these days.

I really feel that simplicity is often overlooked when it comes to flavor. Take for example the simple mix of "East Meets West" Alderwood Smoked Salt and Szechuan Peppercorn Rub (page 9). Smokey, biting, yet pleasingly tingly, it is quite a wonderful taste blast! Many of these recipes evoke a pleasant memory or association. Persian Sumac and Cracked Peppercorn Marinade was introduced to me by my old college roommate. He is Iranian and gave me true appreciation of this inherently healthful and ancient cuisine. Making it brings me back to the Greek islands, where it is slathered on everything from fresh-caught fish and octopus, to zucchini and eggplant. Versatile and amazingly simple, it can be a dressing, marinade, or sandwich topper.

How much is enough? The most common question many cooks ask is how long do you have to marinate something in order to impart flavor. All recipes seem to say 20 minutes minimum to overnight. This is all true; however, overnight marinating achieves the best flavor and needs just a little advance planning. This pretty much sums up the mission here and empowers you to get the best flavor from your grilled items with the least amount of kitchen time. Just rub, soak, and then savor the flavor!

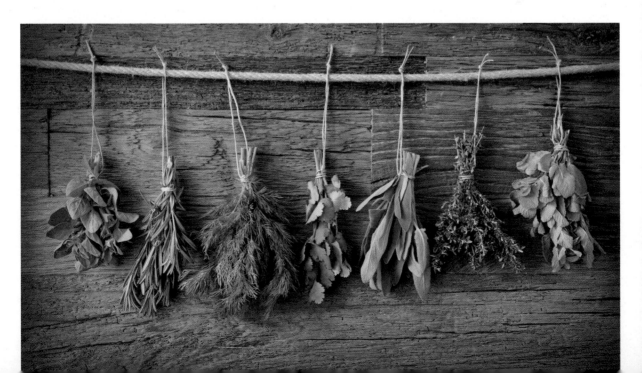

MADRAS CURRY MARINADE

SERVES: 16   **SERVING SIZE:** 1 tablespoon

Spectacular flavor for tofu, tempeh, vegetables, or any protein, this marinade is spicy, tart, and makes any item stand out. I especially like this marinade with tofu grilled and then served over aromatic basmati rice.

- 1/4 cup canola or peanut oil
- 1 tablespoon ginger root, freshly minced
- 3 cloves garlic, minced
- 2 tablespoons curry powder
- 2 tablespoons reduced-sodium soy sauce
- 1/2 cup pineapple juice
- 2 teaspoons red chili flakes

1. Combine all ingredients in a food processor or blender and process for 30 seconds until combined well.

EXCHANGES
1 FAT

CALORIES 40
  CALORIES FROM FAT 30
TOTAL FAT 3.5 g
  SATURATED FAT 0.3 g
  TRANS FAT 0.0 g
CHOLESTEROL 0 mg
SODIUM 70 mg
POTASSIUM 30 mg
TOTAL CARBOHYDRATE 2 g
  DIETARY FIBER 0 g
  SUGARS 1 g
PROTEIN 0 g
PHOSPHORUS 5 mg

TUSCAN LEMON AND ROSEMARY RUB

SERVES: 16   **SERVING SIZE:** 1 tablespoon

This recipe is the foundation of so many regional Italian dishes. The simplicity is brilliant and the flavor is pure. You can substitute any herbs for the rosemary if you prefer.

- 1/2 cup good-quality extra virgin olive oil
- 1/4 cup lemon juice
- 1 tablespoon fresh minced rosemary
- 1/2 teaspoon crushed red chili flakes
- 1 tablespoon chopped fresh parsley

1. Combine all ingredients in a food processor or blender and process for 30 seconds until combined well.

EXCHANGES
1 1/2 FAT

CALORIES 60
  CALORIES FROM FAT 65
TOTAL FAT 7.0 g
  SATURATED FAT 0.9 g
  TRANS FAT 0.0 g
CHOLESTEROL 0 mg
SODIUM 0 mg
POTASSIUM 5 mg
TOTAL CARBOHYDRATE 0 g
  DIETARY FIBER 0 g
  SUGARS 0 g
PROTEIN 0 g
PHOSPHORUS 0 mg

"EAST MEETS WEST" ALDERWOOD SMOKED SALT AND SZECHUAN PEPPERCORN RUB

SERVES: 24　**SERVING SIZE**: 1 teaspoon

This is a unique spice blend that successfully combines flavors from different worlds. Smoky and spicy with a sweet flavor from the anise found in Asian five-spice powder. It's great on anything, especially eggplant and squash.

- 2 teaspoons smoked salt
- 10 teaspoons Szechwuan peppercorns crushed
- 2 tablespoons black peppercorns
- 4 teaspoons granulated garlic
- 2 teaspoons smoked paprika
- 2 teaspoons Asian five-spice powder

1. Combine all ingredients well in a small bowl.

EXCHANGES
FREE FOOD

CALORIES 5
  CALORIES FROM FAT 00
TOTAL FAT 0.0 g
  SATURATED FAT 0.0 g
  TRANS FAT 0.0 g
CHOLESTEROL 0 mg
SODIUM 195 mg
POTASSIUM 30 mg
TOTAL CARBOHYDRATE 2 g
  DIETARY FIBER 1 g
  SUGARS 0 g
PROTEIN 0 g
PHOSPHORUS 5 mg

ATHENIAN GARLIC AND OREGANO DRIZZLE

SERVES: 24　**SERVING SIZE**: 1 tablespoon

In every hidden corner of Greece, this is the go-to marinade for protein from land or sea. It is also incredible on eggplant, zucchini, tomatoes, or feta cheese. I also love it tossed into pasta, rice, or as a crudité dip.

- 1/2 cup extra virgin olive oil
- 1/2 cup lemon juice (about 4 lemons)
- 2 tablespoons fresh chopped oregano
- 2 tablespoons fresh chopped parsley
- 4 cloves minced garlic
- 1 teaspoon ground black pepper

1. Combine all ingredients well in a small bowl.

EXCHANGES
1 FAT

CALORIES 40
  CALORIES FROM FAT 40
TOTAL FAT 4.5 g
  SATURATED FAT 0.6 g
  TRANS FAT 0.0 g
CHOLESTEROL 0 mg
SODIUM 0 mg
POTASSIUM 10 mg
TOTAL CARBOHYDRATE 1 g
  DIETARY FIBER 0 g
  SUGARS 0 g
PROTEIN 0 g
PHOSPHORUS 0 mg

MONSTER MASH

SERVES: 24   SERVING SIZE: 1 tablespoon

I lovingly call this mixture Monster Mash because it's full of wild, intense flavors. I use lemon grass from my garden, but you can find fresh lemon grass in Asian stores. Only use the bottom 3–4 inches of the stalk including the bulb; discard the remainder when making this mash. Or use 2 teaspoons dried lemon grass as a substitute for the fresh. Brush this mixture on skewered vegetables, vegetable steaks, tofu, or tempeh when grilling.

10 peeled cloves garlic
 1 (2-inch) piece unpeeled ginger root
 2 (3-inch) trimmed stalks lemon grass
 1 seeded jalapeno pepper
 ½ cup canola or olive oil

1. In a food processor fitted with the metal blade, combine all ingredients and process until smooth. Refrigerate in a covered container. It will keep for a month.

EXCHANGES
1 FAT

CALORIES 45
  CALORIES FROM FAT 40
TOTAL FAT 4.5 g
  SATURATED FAT 0.3 g
  TRANS FAT 0.0 g
CHOLESTEROL 0 mg
SODIUM 0 mg
POTASSIUM 25 mg
TOTAL CARBOHYDRATE 1 g
  DIETARY FIBER 0 g
  SUGARS 0 g
PROTEIN 0 g
PHOSPHORUS 0 mg

ASIAN FIVE-SPICE MARINADE

SERVES: 32   SERVING SIZE: 1 tablespoon

Five-spice powder can be found in Asian markets and gourmet stores. It is usually a mixture of peppercorns, cinnamon, cloves, star anise, and fennel seeds. This marinade is wonderful on brochettes, eggplant steak, and whole ears of corn.

 1 tablespoon five-spice powder
 ½ cup soy sauce or tamari
 ¼ cup Asian sesame oil
 2 tablespoons Monster Mash (above)
 ¼ cup rice vinegar
 ½ cup pineapple juice or ginger ale

1. In a large mixing bowl, combine all ingredients. Refrigerate in a covered container. It will keep for a month.

EXCHANGES
½ FAT

CALORIES 20
  CALORIES FROM FAT 20
TOTAL FAT 2.0 g
  SATURATED FAT 0.3 g
  TRANS FAT 0.0 g
CHOLESTEROL 0 mg
SODIUM 225 mg
POTASSIUM 15 mg
TOTAL CARBOHYDRATE 1 g
  DIETARY FIBER 0 g
  SUGARS 1 g
PROTEIN 0 g
PHOSPHORUS 5 mg

SOUTH FLORIDA DRY SPICE RUB

SERVES: 60 **SERVING SIZE:** 1 teaspoon

Use this mixture on vegetable steaks, brochettes, ears of corn, tofu steaks, or just about anything. Rub a few teaspoons onto the surface of food after spraying or rubbing it with a bit of oil to help the powder adhere.

¼ cup ground cumin

¼ cup curry powder

¼ cup ground chili powder

2 tablespoons leaf oregano

2 tablespoons freshly ground black pepper

1 tablespoon ground ginger

¼ cup kosher salt

1. Combine all ingredients into a glass mason jar. You can keep this mixture on your pantry shelf forever.

EXCHANGES
FREE FOOD

CALORIES 5
  CALORIES FROM FAT 00
TOTAL FAT 0.0 g
  SATURATED FAT 0.0 g
  TRANS FAT 0.0 g
CHOLESTEROL 0 mg
SODIUM 390 mg
POTASSIUM 30 mg
TOTAL CARBOHYDRATE 1 g
  DIETARY FIBER 0 g
  SUGARS 0 g
PROTEIN 0 g
PHOSPHORUS 5 mg

STEVE'S LATIN BASTE

SERVES: 32 **SERVING SIZE:** 1 tablespoon

Sour orange juice and chilis in adobo can be found in supermarkets, Hispanic markets, and specialty food stores. I love this on whole ears of shucked corn that are basted while grilling.

½ cup sour orange juice

1 cup pineapple juice

1 chipotle chili in adobo

2 tablespoons lime juice

2 tablespoons minced cilantro

1 minced clove garlic

1. In a food processor fitted with the metal blade, combine all ingredients. Process until smooth. Refrigerate in a covered container. It will keep for a month.

EXCHANGES
FREE FOOD

CALORIES 5
  CALORIES FROM FAT 00
TOTAL FAT 0.0 g
  SATURATED FAT 0.0 g
  TRANS FAT 0.0 g
CHOLESTEROL 0 mg
SODIUM 0 mg
POTASSIUM 20 mg
TOTAL CARBOHYDRATE 2 g
  DIETARY FIBER 0 g
  SUGARS 1 g
PROTEIN 0 g
PHOSPHORUS 0 mg

DUKKAH SPICE SPRINKLE

SERVES: 24   **SERVING SIZE:** 1 tablespoon

There are many version of this nut, seed, and spice mixture originating in Egypt. You can combine it with a drizzle of extra virgin olive oil, but lately I've been putting it over pasta, legumes, rice, and sautéed vegetables and I'm hooked. I'd like to say that I can stop anytime… but I can't. The key to this recipe is toasting the nuts in the oven and spices in a dry pan to release the aromatic tastes.

³/₄ cup almonds, hazelnuts, or macadamia nuts
1 teaspoon fennel seeds
1 teaspoon anise seeds
1 tablespoon cumin seeds
2 tablespoons coriander seeds
¹/₂ cup sesame seeds
1 teaspoon sea salt
1 tablespoon cracked black peppercorns

1. Preheat the oven to 300°F. Place the nuts on a baking pan in the oven and toast for approximately 15 minutes until lightly browned. Watch carefully as they burn easily. Set aside. If using whole-skin-on nuts, place them in a kitchen towel and rub together to remove skins.

2. Heat a medium sauté pan over moderate heat and add the fennel seeds, anise seeds, cumin seeds, coriander seeds, and sesame seeds. Heat the spices in the dry pan, stirring constantly, for 2–3 minutes until they become very fragrant and begin to color. Remove from the pan and pour into a bowl.

3. Place all ingredients including salt and pepper in a food processor fitted with a standard S blade and process until ground but with small pieces.

4. Keep in a small covered jar in a cool place.

EXCHANGES
1 FAT

CALORIES 45
  CALORIES FROM FAT 35
TOTAL FAT 4.0 g
  SATURATED FAT 0.4 g
  TRANS FAT 0.0 g
CHOLESTEROL 0 mg
SODIUM 90 mg
POTASSIUM 65 mg
TOTAL CARBOHYDRATE 2 g
  DIETARY FIBER 1 g
  SUGARS 0 g
PROTEIN 2 g
PHOSPHORUS 45 mg

GOLD RUSH YOGURT LEMON DILL MARINADE

SERVES: 4   **SERVING SIZE**: 1/2 cup

This is an incredible marinade for chicken, seafood, pork, or lamb. The enzymes in the yogurt act as a tenderizer and permeate with immense flavor. You may use curry, annatto, or turmeric for the yellow color.

- 1 cup plain fat-free Greek yogurt
- 2 teaspoons turmeric, ground
- 1/4 cup fresh dill, minced
- 1/4 cup red onion, minced
- 2 tablespoons extra virgin olive oil
  Juice of 1 lemon
- 1 teaspoon black pepper, ground

1. Combine all ingredients in a small mixing bowl. Toss in your favorite protein, cover, and marinate at least 1 hour or overnight in the refrigerator, turning occasionally.

EXCHANGES
1/2 FAT-FREE MILK
1 FAT

CALORIES 105
  CALORIES FROM FAT 65
TOTAL FAT 7.0 g
  SATURATED FAT 1.0 g
  TRANS FAT 0.0 g
CHOLESTEROL 0 mg
SODIUM 25 mg
POTASSIUM 130 mg
TOTAL CARBOHYDRATE 5 g
  DIETARY FIBER 1 g
  SUGARS 3 g
PROTEIN 6 g
PHOSPHORUS 85 mg

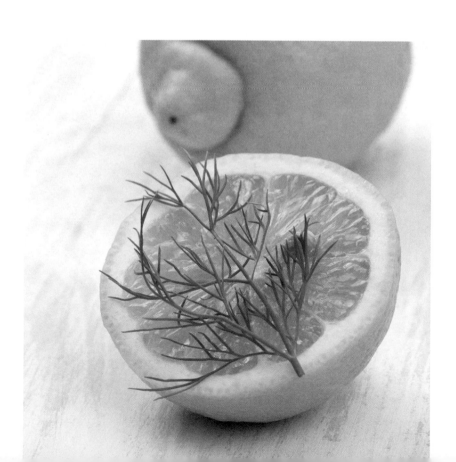

FIRE AND ICE CHIPOTLE MINT MARINADE

SERVES: 6   **SERVING SIZE**: 1/6 recipe

What a tease to your taste buds. Fiery chipotle chilis smack you in the face first then the fresh cooling mint takes over. I love this on chicken or pork, although I've had friends use it on duck and turkey before the meat hits the grill.

2 chipotle chilis en adobo

2 tablespoons liquid from the canned chipotle chili

1/2 cup lime juice

2 tablespoons extra virgin olive oil

1–1 1/2 tablespoons agave or honey

1/4 cup fresh mint, chopped

1. Combine all ingredients in a food processor or blender and puree for 30 seconds until well combined and smooth.

2. Place your favorite protein in a large plastic bag and pour in the marinade. Massage the marinade into the protein, place in refrigerator, and allow to marinate at least 30 minutes, or for best results, overnight.

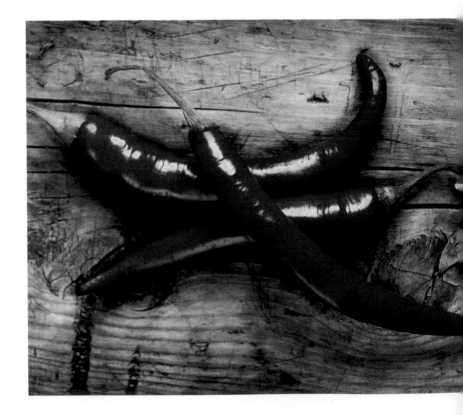

EXCHANGES
1/2 CARBOHYDRATE
1 FAT

CALORIES 65
  CALORIES FROM FAT 45
TOTAL FAT 5.0 g
  SATURATED FAT 0.6 g
  TRANS FAT 0.0 g
CHOLESTEROL 0 mg
SODIUM 55 mg
POTASSIUM 45 mg
TOTAL CARBOHYDRATE 6 g
  DIETARY FIBER 1 g
  SUGARS 4 g
PROTEIN 0 g
PHOSPHORUS 5 mg

GREEN THAI CURRY BLAST MARINADE

SERVES: 6 **SERVING SIZE**: ¹/₆ recipe

I love the intense spice of Thai food. From tart lime, to spicy chili peppers, fresh cilantro, and lemongrass, my mouth is so happy when these flavors meet. Thai green curry paste and fish sauce are available in all Asian markets and many supermarkets.

3 tablespoons Thai green curry paste

1²/₃ cups unsweetened almond milk or water

2 tablespoons lime juice

2 teaspoons fish sauce or reduced-sodium soy sauce

¹/₄ cup scallions, minced

¹/₄ cup cilantro, minced

1 tablespoon agave

1. Combine all ingredients in a food processor or blender and purée for 30 seconds until well combined and smooth.

2. Place your favorite protein in a large plastic bag and pour in the marinade. Massage the marinade into the protein, place in refrigerator, and allow to marinate at least 30 minutes, or for best results, overnight.

EXCHANGES
¹/₂ CARBOHYDRATE

CALORIES 25
  CALORIES FROM FAT 5
TOTAL FAT 0.5 g
  SATURATED FAT 0.0 g
  TRANS FAT 0.0 g
CHOLESTEROL 0 mg
SODIUM 455 mg
POTASSIUM 70 mg
TOTAL CARBOHYDRATE 5 g
  DIETARY FIBER 0 g
  SUGARS 4 g
PROTEIN 0 g
PHOSPHORUS 10 mg

PERSIAN SUMAC AND CRACKED PEPPERCORN MARINADE

SERVES: 6   **SERVING SIZE**: ¹/₆ recipe

Persian food is inherently healthy. My roommate through college was Persian and taught me how to cook many staple dishes. I developed a love for sumac, a lemony tasting, ruby-colored ground dried berry that gives everything a wonderful tart taste. It's amazing on burgers, lamb, or grilled eggplant as well. You can find it in Middle Eastern stores or order it online.

2 tablespoons ground sumac

3 tablespoons extra virgin olive oil

¹/₄ cup flat leaf parsley, chopped

¹/₂ onion, chopped

2 cloves garlic, minced

Juice of 1 lime

1 teaspoon black pepper, ground

1. Combine all ingredients in a food processor or blender and purée for 30 seconds until well combined and smooth.

2. Place your favorite protein in a large plastic bag and pour in the marinade. Massage the marinade into the protein, place in refrigerator, and allow to marinate at least 30 minutes, or for best results, overnight.

EXCHANGES
1¹/₂ FAT

CALORIES 75
  CALORIES FROM FAT 65
TOTAL FAT 7.0 g
  SATURATED FAT 0.9 g
  TRANS FAT 0.0 g
CHOLESTEROL 0 mg
SODIUM 5 mg
POTASSIUM 35 mg
TOTAL CARBOHYDRATE 3 g
  DIETARY FIBER 0 g
  SUGARS 1 g
PROTEIN 0 g
PHOSPHORUS 5 mg

BLACK COFFEE MOJO MARINADE

SERVES: 16   **SERVING SIZE**: ¼ cup

Incredible on pork, lamb, or beef. A friend of mine uses this marinade for whole pork butts and fresh hams. You'll get the best results by marinating large cuts of meat overnight in the refrigerator.

2 cups black coffee

1 cup orange juice

¼ cup olive oil

¼ cup white vinegar

1 tablespoon smoked paprika

1 tablespoon ground cumin or seeds

1 tablespoon anise seeds

3 cloves garlic, minced

1 jalapeño, seeded, minced

2 chipotles en adobo, minced

½ cup cilantro, minced

1. Combine all ingredients in a food processor or blender and purée for 30 seconds until well combined and smooth.

2. Place your favorite protein in a large plastic bag and pour in the marinade. Massage the marinade into the protein, place in refrigerator, and allow to marinate at least 30 minutes, or overnight, for best results.

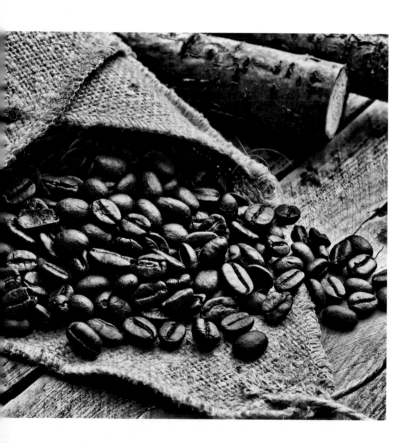

EXCHANGES
1 FAT

CALORIES 45
  CALORIES FROM FAT 30
TOTAL FAT 3.5 g
  SATURATED FAT 0.5 g
  TRANS FAT 0.0 g
CHOLESTEROL 0 mg
SODIUM 10 mg
POTASSIUM 80 mg
TOTAL CARBOHYDRATE 3 g
  DIETARY FIBER 0 g
  SUGARS 2 g
PROTEIN 0 g
PHOSPHORUS 10 mg

CHAPTER 2
Center of the Plate

How we eat has changed significantly since I was a kid. Today, it seems that anyone who loves food is enamored with global cuisine and recipes. International food options or unusual ingredients are now readily available in large supermarkets across the country.

I love this, by the way. I've included a huge selection of entrée items from every protein category. Whether you love a juicy steak or a slab of grilled tofu, these recipes all reflect my love of food. I felt it was important to include recipes from my many travels across the globe. I'm fascinated by what people around the world eat and cook for their families. I've had the good fortune to cook family recipes alongside grandmas in ancient Greece, monks in monasteries in the mountains of obscure Mediterranean islands, and everyday people in small towns across our own food-rich country. This is what makes up the collection of recipes that you'll find within this chapter. I think

grilling is fun and relaxing and I've tried to emphasize recipes that are not typical, yet remain easy to prepare. From Peruvian chicken that melts in your mouth, to food on sticks, wrapped in leaves and foil, and some of the best burgers you will ever eat, I think you'll love grilling the way I do once you sample a few of the recipes in this chapter.

Most of these center of the plate recipes were derived from meaningful culinary experiences. It makes me realize that even though the recipe may be simple in ingredients and method, it remains a powerful and memorable eating event. When you make the Jamaican Stuffed Fish with Ritz (page 43), I think your taste buds will be awakened and appreciate the fact that this dish is extraordinarily simple, flavorful, and satisfying. My intention is to create go-to grill recipes for you to experiment with, doctor to your own liking, and carry forward to your family and friends.

PERUVIAN SUPER CHICKEN

SERVES: 6   **SERVING SIZE**: 2 thighs

Peruvian food is becoming more popular here in our country. This version is from a good friend of mine, also a chef. Brining makes the chicken juicy and so tender it's almost falling apart after cooking. This chicken is amazing in wraps, on salads, in burritos, or over rice.

RINSE
- 1 quart cold water
- ½ cup lime juice
- 2 pounds (about 12 thighs) boneless skinless chicken thighs

PERUVIAN MARINADE
- ½ cup white wine
- ¼ cup olive oil
- ⅓ cup reduced-sodium soy sauce
- 4 cloves minced garlic
- 1 tablespoon cumin
- 1 tablespoon paprika
- 1 tablespoon oregano

1. Combine cold water and lime juice in bowl. Soak the chicken in the mixture for 20 minutes. Rinse off chicken and transfer to a large plastic bag.

2. Combine the Peruvian Marinade ingredients in a medium mixing bowl and pour over chicken in a large sealable plastic bag. Massage the marinade over the chicken and marinate at least 2 hours or overnight, if possible.

3. Grill chicken following our grill recommendations or covered in a 350°F oven for 35 minutes in its own juice. Uncover and continue to cook for an additional 15 minutes until cooked through and lightly browned.

EXCHANGES
4 LEAN MEAT
1 FAT

CALORIES 235
  CALORIES FROM FAT 115
TOTAL FAT 13.0 g
  SATURATED FAT 3.0 g
  TRANS FAT 0.0 g
CHOLESTEROL 135 mg
SODIUM 335 mg
POTASSIUM 325 mg
TOTAL CARBOHYDRATE 2 g
  DIETARY FIBER 0 g
  SUGARS 0 g
PROTEIN 25 g
PHOSPHORUS 235 mg

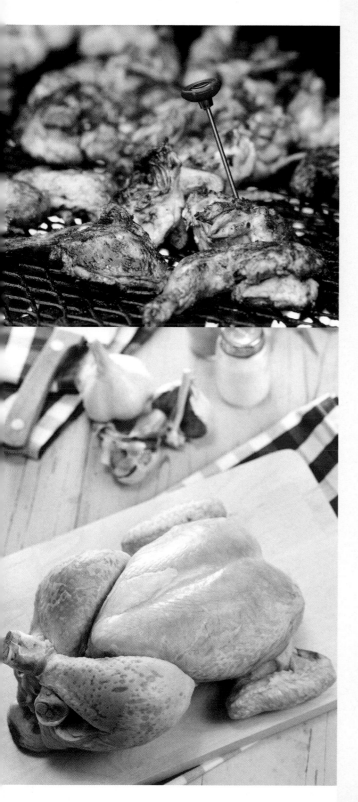

TEST CHICKEN FOR DONENESS

There are a few ways to test any cut of chicken to make sure it is cooked through. Probably the single most awful feeling is biting into chicken that's not cooked properly.

A thermometer is the most effective way of measuring the internal temperature of cooked meat. A thermometer is inserted into the thickest part of the chicken, whether it is the entire chicken or a breast or thigh, and left in and stays inserted throughout the cooking process. Below is a chart of doneness temps.

INTERNAL TEMPERATURES FOR PROPER DONENESS	
Whole Chicken—Thigh Area	175°–180°F
Whole Chicken—Breast Area	170°–175°F
Chicken Breast and Wings	170°–175°F
Chicken Parts—Dark Meat	180°F
Ground Chicken	170°F
Stuffing Inside Whole Chicken	165°F
Note: If the proper temperature is not reached, the chicken should be returned to the heat source for further cooking.	

Instant-read thermometers are inserted into the thickest part of the chicken (don't place it directly against the bone) to read the temperature once the chicken is thought to be cooked. It takes about 10–15 seconds to register the proper temperature.

Visual examination or piercing is another way to test the doneness of the chicken. With a paring knife, skewer, or other sharp object, cut into the thickest part or pierce the chicken to see that the juices run clear. If they are pink, continue to cook the chicken until the juice runs clear. This means it has reached the proper internal temperature and is fully cooked through.

CHIMMI CHURRI BEEF

SERVES: 4   **SERVING SIZE:** ¼ recipe   **MARINATING TIME:** At least 1 hour or overnight

This is such a universal recipe that is delicious whether you use beef, shrimp, tofu, or turkey. I really enjoy the tart combination of vinegar, capers, and spicy jalapeño. I try to keep a jar in my fridge at all times.

CHIMMI CHURRI SAUCE

¼ cup olive oil

¼ cup water

½ cup red wine vinegar

3 cloves garlic, minced

¼ cup capers, drained and rinsed

1 teaspoon oregano

½ cup parsley, fresh minced

½ jalapeño pepper, seeded and minced

½ teaspoon salt

1 pound skirt steak, flank steak, or top sirloin, trimmed of excess fat

1. Make the Chimmi Churri Sauce. There will be enough to both marinate the skewers and use as a sauce after grilling. Combine the olive oil, vinegar, garlic, capers, oregano, parsley, jalapeño pepper, and salt in a food processor or blender and purée until smooth. Set aside and measure out ½ cup for marinating steak.

2. Pour the ½ cup of Chimmi Churri Sauce over the beef and marinate for at least 1 hour or preferably overnight in the refrigerator, turning occasionally. Discard leftover marinade.

3. Grill the steak over a moderately hot grill for 4–6 minutes, turn over and repeat until cooked through.

4. Serve skewers with remaining Chimmi Churri Sauce.

EXCHANGES
1 VEGETABLE
3 LEAN MEAT
2 FAT

CALORIES 270
  CALORIES FROM FAT 145
TOTAL FAT 16.0 g
  SATURATED FAT 3.9 g
  TRANS FAT 0.0 g
CHOLESTEROL 60 mg
SODIUM 465 mg
POTASSIUM 430 mg
TOTAL CARBOHYDRATE 7 g
  DIETARY FIBER 1 g
  SUGARS 4 g
PROTEIN 23 g
PHOSPHORUS 200 mg

FOR CHIMMI CHURRI
SAUCE ONLY (SERVING SIZE:
1 TABLESPOON)

EXCHANGES
1 FAT

CALORIES 35
  CALORIES FROM FAT 30
TOTAL FAT 3.5 G
  SATURATED FAT 0.5 G
  TRANS FAT 0.0 G
CHOLESTEROL 0 MG
SODIUM 140 MG
POTASSIUM 25 MG
TOTAL CARBOHYDRATE 1 G
  DIETARY FIBER 0 G
  SUGARS 0 G
PROTEIN 0 G
PHOSPHORUS 0 MG

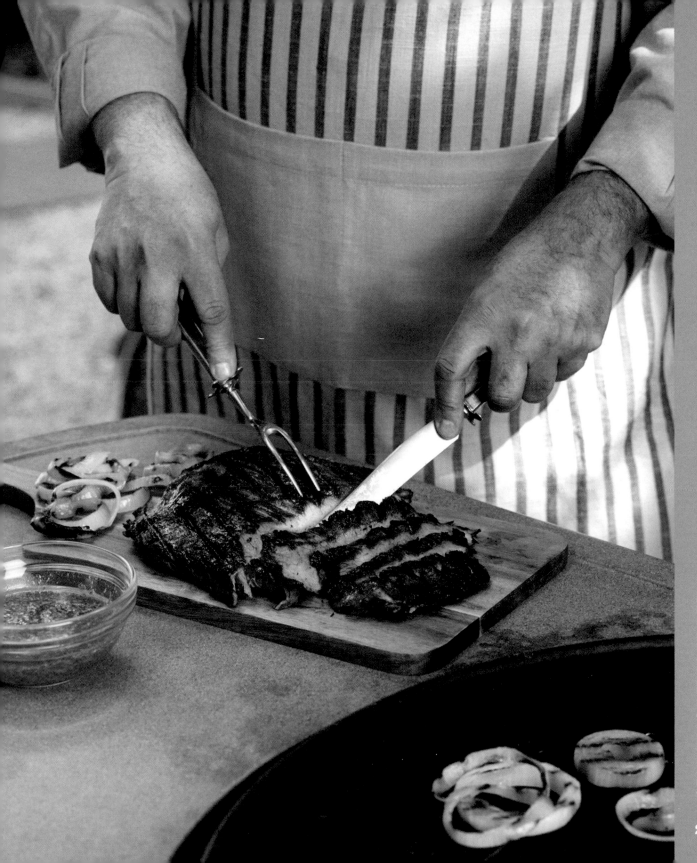

FLATTENED CORNISH HENS WITH CRACKED CUMIN AND CHIPOTLE CRUST

SERVES: 4   **SERVING SIZE**: 1 hen   **MARINATING TIME**: At least 30 minutes or overnight

Although this recipe takes a bit of time to prep, it creates the 'wow' factor when you are having guests over for a cookout. It comes from a classic grilling technique where chicken is cooked under the weight of a heavy brick. This flattens the meat and creates an even surface that sears the meat evenly, producing a crispy caramelized surface and juicy moist result below the skin. Here we give it a strong Southwest flavor of smoky chipotle chilies and cumin seed.

CHIPOTLE MARINADE

2 tablespoons olive oil
  Juice of 2 limes (about 2 tablespoons)
1 tablespoon crushed cumin seeds (you can use ground, but cracked whole seeds taste better)
2 cloves garlic, minced
2 chipotle chilies en adobo, minced
1 teaspoon smoked paprika

4 Cornish hens, backbone removed and flattened
4 bricks wrapped in aluminum foil

1. Combine all of the Chipotle Marinade ingredients in a small bowl. Transfer marinade into a large, tightly sealed plastic bag and add Cornish hens. Massage the marinade into the Cornish hens well. Marinate at least 30 minutes at room temperature or overnight in the refrigerator. Discard marinade before grilling.

2. Preheat grill to medium-high heat and place Cornish hens on grill grate. Cook as per directions for indirect heat method (page 3). Place the foil-wrapped brick on top of the Cornish hen and press down gently. Continue to cook over medium-low heat for approximately 20–23 minutes per side, replacing the brick when turned until cooked through.

EXCHANGES
6 LEAN MEAT

CALORIES 295
  CALORIES FROM FAT 100
TOTAL FAT 11.0 g
  SATURATED FAT 2.4 g
  TRANS FAT 0.0 g
CHOLESTEROL 205 mg
SODIUM 150 mg
POTASSIUM 515 mg
TOTAL CARBOHYDRATE 2 g
  DIETARY FIBER 0 g
  SUGARS 0 g
PROTEIN 45 g
PHOSPHORUS 295 mg

MISO MUSTARD SHRIMP AND GREEN ONION STICKS

SERVES: 4 **SERVING SIZE:** ¼ recipe **MARINATING TIME:** At least 15 minutes

Although most of us are familiar with miso because of Japanese miso soup, it is an incredible ingredient to add to many recipes. I favor the delicate slightly sweet taste of white miso, but there are several other varieties. The darker the color, the more intense the flavor. White goes well with shrimp and allows the seafood and grill flavors to blend well.

MARINADE

- 1 tablespoon olive oil
- 2 tablespoons Dijon-style mustard
- 1 tablespoon stone-ground mustard with seeds
- 1 tablespoon honey
- 1 tablespoon white miso
  Juice of 1 orange
  Juice of 1 lemon

- 1 pound medium to large shrimp, peeled and deveined, tail on or off
- 2 bunches scallions, root ends trimmed, cut into 2-inch lengths
- 10–12 wooden or metal skewers

1. Combine all of the marinade ingredients in a small bowl, then pour into a large tightly sealed plastic bag with shrimp. Marinate at least 15 minutes at room temperature for best results.

2. Preheat grill to medium-high heat. Thread shrimp and green onion sections on skewers, alternating shrimp and green onions.

3. Place skewers on grill grate. Cook as per directions for direct heat method (page 3), keeping in mind that shrimp cook very quickly and 3-4 minutes per side should be enough to cook the skewers through to opaque.

EXCHANGES
½ CARBOHYDRATE
3 LEAN MEAT

CALORIES 140
  CALORIES FROM FAT 20
TOTAL FAT 2.5 g
  SATURATED FAT 0.3 g
  TRANS FAT 0.0 g
CHOLESTEROL 190 mg
SODIUM 275 mg
POTASSIUM 320 mg
TOTAL CARBOHYDRATE 6 g
  DIETARY FIBER 1 g
  SUGARS 4 g
PROTEIN 25 g
PHOSPHORUS 250 mg

ON GRILLING SEAFOOD

The most delicate of all grilled foods, seafood is simply incredible when cooked correctly. However, the difference between cooked and overcooked when it comes to seafood can be a matter of 30 seconds. When cooking seafood, you really need to focus for no more than 10 minutes at most on the task at hand. I always cook fresh steaks on high heat to sear in the juice, I turn the seafood only once to sear the other side, and then move it to a cooler area of the grill for a few minutes to cook through while keeping juicy. I constantly baste the fish with a marinade while cooking and pull it from the grill when it just turns opaque. You should try grilling a whole fish at least once, because it is such an amazing way to enjoy seafood. I simply score the fish in a crosshatch fashion, marinate it in one of our marinade recipes or a dry rub and cook it through using direct heat method (page 3). The bones of the whole fish act as serious heat conductors and help cook the fish through in a matter of minutes. You'll know when it's done, because the meat lifts off away from the bones easily.

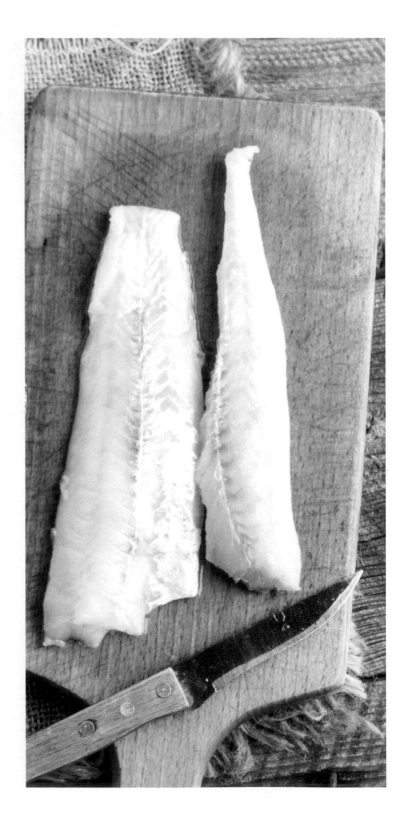

CHEFS SURPRISE GRILLED SEAFOOD PACKAGES

SERVES: 4   **SERVING SIZE**: ¹/₄ recipe

Delicate seafood, crisp vegetables, and fresh herbs pick up the flavor of the grill inside these wonderful little packages. The steam generated inside the foil produces intense flavors. Serve the packets with a bold sauce or relish. Try the Chimmi Churri Sauce (page 89). I like to add a few slices of raw jalapeño or Serrano chili pepper to give the dish a little extra spiciness.

- 4 fish filets (about 6 ounces each), such as mahi mahi, flounder, haddock, sole, or cod
- ¹/₂ cup onions or leeks, thinly sliced
- ¹/₄ cup carrots, thinly sliced or julienned
- ¹/₄ cup celery, thinly sliced
- 1 cup spinach leaves
- 4 whole sprigs of fresh herbs left on the branch, such as thyme, basil, tarragon, or oregano
- ¹/₄ cup dry white wine, such as Sauvignon Blanc, Chardonnay, or Dry Riesling
- 4 teaspoons of no–trans–fat nonhydrogenated buttery spread (such as Smart Balance)
- ¹/₂ teaspoon kosher salt
- 4 pieces aluminum foil in 12-inch squares

1. Place the 4 pieces of foil on a work surface in front of you. On each, place a fish filet and divide the vegetables, herbs, wine, and butter over the fish. Seal the packages well.

2. Preheat the grill to medium-high heat and place the packets on the grill.

3. Cook as per directions for direct heat (page 3) for approximately 12–15 minutes until fish is cooked through and vegetables are tender.

4. Serve immediately, making sure to open the packets in front of each guest so they can inhale the incredible aromatic results of your work. Be careful when opening the packets because of the steam.

EXCHANGES
4 LEAN MEAT

CALORIES 190
  CALORIES FROM FAT 40
TOTAL FAT 4.5 g
  SATURATED FAT 1.2 g
  TRANS FAT 0.0 g
CHOLESTEROL 125 mg
SODIUM 430 mg
POTASSIUM 820 mg
TOTAL CARBOHYDRATE 3 g
  DIETARY FIBER 1 g
  SUGARS 1 g
PROTEIN 32 g
PHOSPHORUS 255 mg

GRILLED ATHENIAN BURGER

SERVES: 4   **SERVING SIZE:** 1 burger

When is a burger not just a burger? You'll soon find out after trying this version. You may substitute 50% lamb for beef in this recipe as well. I sometimes spike this recipe with crushed red chili flakes or a minced Serrano chili because I'm a spicy food freak.

1 pound 95% lean ground beef
4 tablespoons fat-free Greek yogurt
1 clove minced garlic
1 teaspoon leaf oregano
2 tablespoons fresh leaf parsley, chopped
1/2 teaspoon lemon zest (lemon peel, grated)
1/4 teaspoon ground black pepper

1. In a large mixing bowl combine all ingredients and mix until just combined.

2. Divide mixture into 4 equal parts and form 4 burgers. Place on a plate and refrigerate until ready for grilling.

3. Spray grill or stove-top grill pan with high-heat olive or canola oil spray. Heat grill to high temperature (450–500°F).

4. Grill burgers for approximately 6–8 minutes. Turn and repeat process for an additional 4–5 minutes. Check for doneness with a thermometer. Internal temperature should be about 160°F as they will continue to cook for a few minutes.

5. Serve with Greek Yogurt Spread (below). Top with fresh romaine leaves, sliced tomatoes, and red onion on a whole-grain bun or wrapped in a pita.

FOR GRILLED ATHENIAN BURGER	FOR GREEK YOGURT SPREAD
EXCHANGES 4 LEAN MEAT	**EXCHANGES** FREE FOOD
CALORIES 160 **CALORIES FROM FAT** 55	**CALORIES** 20 **CALORIES FROM FAT** 00
TOTAL FAT 6.0 g **SATURATED FAT** 2.7 g **TRANS FAT** 0.1 g	**TOTAL FAT** 0.0 g **SATURATED FAT** 0.0 g **TRANS FAT** 0.0 g
CHOLESTEROL 70 mg	**CHOLESTEROL** 0 mg
SODIUM 70 mg	**SODIUM** 290 mg
POTASSIUM 390 mg	**POTASSIUM** 35 mg
TOTAL CARBOHYDRATE 1 g **DIETARY FIBER** 0 g **SUGARS** 1 g	**TOTAL CARBOHYDRATE** 2 g **DIETARY FIBER** 0 g **SUGARS** 1 g
PROTEIN 24 g	**PROTEIN** 3 g
PHOSPHORUS 225 mg	**PHOSPHORUS** 40 mg

GREEK YOGURT SPREAD

SERVES: 8   **SERVING SIZE:** 2 tablespoons

This simple Greek yogurt spread is incredible over a burger, grilled chicken skewers, or grilled vegetables. I add 1/2 cup of grated, peeled cucumber for a cooling addition.

1 cup fat-free Greek yogurt
1 tablespoon Montreal steak seasoning (spicy or regular)
1/4 cup chopped parsley or mint
2 tablespoons crumbled feta cheese

1. In a small bowl, combine all ingredients and mix well.

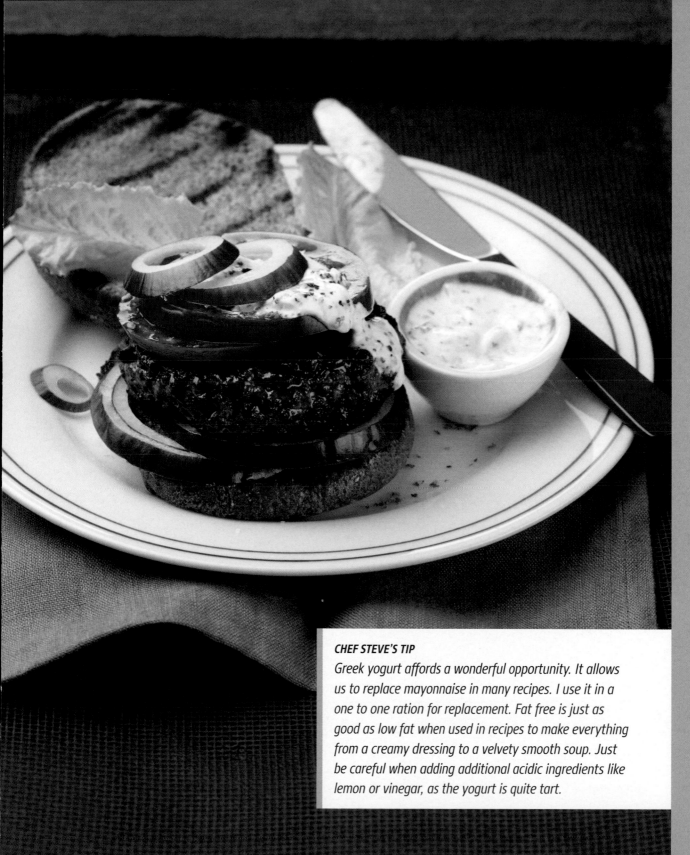

CHEF STEVE'S TIP

Greek yogurt affords a wonderful opportunity. It allows us to replace mayonnaise in many recipes. I use it in a one to one ration for replacement. Fat free is just as good as low fat when used in recipes to make everything from a creamy dressing to a velvety smooth soup. Just be careful when adding additional acidic ingredients like lemon or vinegar, as the yogurt is quite tart.

AROMATIC TEA AND GINGER MARINATED CHICKEN BREAST

SERVES: 8   **SERVING SIZE**: 1 breast   **MARINATING TIME**: Overnight

The use of tea in this recipe adds an incredible smoky, sweet flavor and wonderful aroma. Try it for marinating pork and lamb as well. If you like over-the-top flavor, add 2 whole star anise buds found in all Asian markets.

4 cups water, divided use

4 tea bags of your favorite flavor (I recommend Oolong)

1 cinnamon stick

2 bay leaves

1 heaping tablespoon minced fresh ginger root

2 cloves garlic, chopped

2 tablespoons brown sugar

1 tablespoon reduced-sodium soy sauce

1 tablespoon coarsely ground black pepper

1 whole chicken or 8 chicken legs and 8 chicken breasts

1. Boil 2 cups of water. Add all the ingredients except chicken. Steep for 10 minutes off the heat. Add the remaining 2 cups of water and cool.

2. Score the chicken through the skin with a sharp knife, making cuts about ¼-inch deep.

3. Add the cooled marinade to the chicken in a large pan and refrigerate overnight for best flavor.

4. Drain and pat well. Cook chicken either on grill, in a grill pan, under the broiler, or in a sauté pan until cooked through.

EXCHANGES
5 LEAN MEAT

CALORIES 200
 CALORIES FROM FAT 35
TOTAL FAT 4.0 g
 SATURATED FAT 1.2 g
 TRANS FAT 0.0 g
CHOLESTEROL 100 mg
SODIUM 125 mg
POTASSIUM 325 mg
TOTAL CARBOHYDRATE 2 g
 DIETARY FIBER 0 g
 SUGARS 2 g
PROTEIN 36 g
PHOSPHORUS 270 mg

LEMON TARRAGON SEARED SALMON WITH KIWI ROMA TOMATO SALSA

SERVES: 4   **SERVING SIZE**: ¼ recipe   **MARINATING TIME**: 10 minutes

This is a delicate way to prepare salmon, which allows the natural flavor of the salmon to peek through. I try to use wild-caught salmon if available as it has so much more flavor, has good fat content, and excellent nutritional benefits.

1 teaspoon olive oil
Juice of 1 lemon
½ teaspoon lemon zest
½ teaspoon minced tarragon
1 teaspoon Dijon-style mustard
16 ounce salmon filet, cut into 4 pieces
2 teaspoons panko (Japanese) breadcrumbs

KIWI SALSA
1 ripe kiwi, peeled and diced into ½-inch squares
1 ripe Roma tomato, diced into ½-inch squares
1 tablespoon red onion, minced
1 teaspoon jalapeño or serrano chili, minced
1 tablespoon flat leaf parsley, minced
Juice of ½ lime
1 teaspoon extra virgin olive oil

1. Combine oil, lemon juice, lemon zest, tarragon, and mustard in a small mixing bowl.

2. Marinate salmon filets in marinade for 10 minutes. Remove from marinade and press lightly into Panko breadcrumbs.

3. Heat a grill pan or gas grill over medium-high heat and place salmon into pan or heated char grill grate. Sear salmon for 3–4 minutes. Turn salmon and repeat process. Move salmon to a cooler part of the grill and continue to cook for 4–6 minutes until fully cooked through.

4. Make Kiwi Salsa by combining all ingredients in a medium mixing bowl. Serve over salmon filets.

EXCHANGES
½ CARBOHYDRATE
4 LEAN MEAT
1 FAT

CALORIES 240
  CALORIES FROM FAT 115
TOTAL FAT 13.0 g
  SATURATED FAT 2.1 g
  TRANS FAT 0.0 g
CHOLESTEROL 80 mg
SODIUM 95 mg
POTASSIUM 470 mg
TOTAL CARBOHYDRATE 5 g
  DIETARY FIBER 1 g
  SUGARS 3 g
PROTEIN 26 g
PHOSPHORUS 270 mg

ROASTED RED PEPPER TOFU STEAKS WITH AVOCADO LIME SALSA

SERVES: 2   **SERVING SIZE**: 1/2 recipe   **MARINATING TIME**: At least 1 hour or overnight

There are dozens of red pepper pastes available in all Asian markets. Thai, Korean, and Chinese varieties are all wonderful in this recipe. They are available in both spicy and non-spicy versions. If you prefer, and have the time, use an equal amount of the Quick Red Pepper Paste (recipe below). Tofu is better when marinated overnight, because it absorbs the flavor of the marinade.

1/2 cup red pepper paste
(see recipe below or use packaged)

2 cloves minced garlic

1 tablespoon lower-sodium soy sauce

1 tablespoon lime juice

1 pound firm or extra firm light tofu, cut into 1/2-inch-thick steaks cut across the short side

QUICK RED PEPPER PASTE

1/2 cup jarred roasted red peppers, drained, rinsed, and patted dry.

1 tablespoon tomato paste

2 cloves garlic, minced

1/2 teaspoon crushed red chili flakes

2 teaspoons smoked red pepper paste

1/2 cup olive oil

1. Combine all Quick Red Pepper Paste ingredients (if using recipe) in a food processor, blender, or hand-held immersion blender for 30 seconds until a smooth paste is formed. Combine red pepper paste, garlic, soy sauce, and lime juice in a mixing bowl.

2. Pour over the tofu and rub into the surface. Allow to marinate at least 1 hour in the refrigerator, or for best flavor, overnight.

3. Grill over coals, gas grill, or in a broiler (see our grilling recommendations, page 3).

4. Serve with Avocado Lime Salsa (see right).

FOR 1 SERVING OF TOFU STEAK WITH 2 SERVINGS AVOCADO LIME SALSA

EXCHANGES
1/2 CARBOHYDRATE
3 LEAN MEAT
2 1/2 FAT

CALORIES 275
  CALORIES FROM FAT 170
TOTAL FAT 19.0 g
  SATURATED FAT 2.6 g
  TRANS FAT 0.0 g
CHOLESTEROL 0 mg
SODIUM 545 mg
POTASSIUM 395 mg
TOTAL CARBOHYDRATE 11 g
  DIETARY FIBER 2 g
  SUGARS 4 g
PROTEIN 18 g
PHOSPHORUS 230 mg

AVOCADO LIME SALSA

SERVES: 8   **SERVING SIZE**: ⅛ recipe

This is my "go to" green salsa or Salsa Verde. I use it for almost any grilled item, not because it's simple, but because I really love it. Judging from most people's reactions, they do too. Jarred or canned tomatillos are a good substitute for fresh if you don't have the time to roast fresh tomatillos yourself. Use the chopped or whole tomatillos packed in water.

1 cup chopped tomatillos
½ cup Spanish onion, chopped
2 cloves garlic, minced
1 serrano chili, minced
½ cup cilantro, minced
  Juice of 1 lime
  Salt to taste
1 large avocado, chopped

1. Combine all ingredients well in a medium mixing bowl, making sure to add avocado last.

EXCHANGES
1 FAT

CALORIES 45
  CALORIES FROM FAT 30
TOTAL FAT 3.5 g
  SATURATED FAT 0.5 g
  TRANS FAT 0.0 g
CHOLESTEROL 0 mg
SODIUM 00 mg
POTASSIUM 180 mg
TOTAL CARBOHYDRATE 4 g
  DIETARY FIBER 2 g
  SUGARS 1 g
PROTEIN 1 g
PHOSPHORUS 25 mg

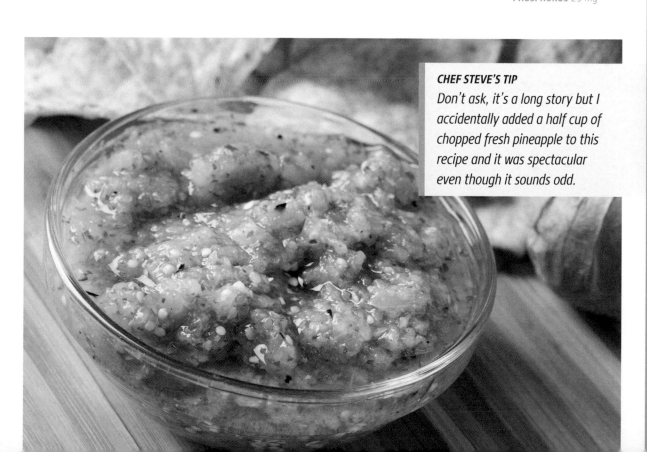

CHEF STEVE'S TIP
Don't ask, it's a long story but I accidentally added a half cup of chopped fresh pineapple to this recipe and it was spectacular even though it sounds odd.

GRILLED DUCK WITH GREEN PEPPERCORN AND TANGERINE

SERVES: 4   **SERVING SIZE:** 1/4 recipe   **MARINATING TIME:** At least 1 hour or overnight

This recipe is worthy of a special occasion meal. You can find frozen duck breasts already boned in many supermarkets or specialty stores. Green peppercorns are spicy, pungent, and bold in flavor, adding a very unusual taste to any protein. They are especially suited to strong meats and poultry.

4 duck breasts, boneless, skin on
1/2 teaspoon kosher or sea salt
Fresh pepper from peppermill

DUCK SAUCE
1/2 cup low-sugar, bitter orange marmalade
Juice of 2 tangerines
1/4 cup white wine or sherry vinegar
1 tablespoon lower-sodium soy sauce
1 tablespoon green peppercorns

1. With a sharp knife, make an incision in the duck breasts about 1/4 inch deep in a crisscross fashion. Season with salt and pepper.

2. Preheat grill to medium-high heat and place on grill grate. Cook as per directions for indirect heat method (page 3). The last 5 minutes of cooking, brush some of the sauce on both sides and allow to caramelize before serving.

3. In the meantime, make the duck sauce. In a medium saucepot, heat orange marmalade, tangerine juice, wine or vinegar, soy sauce, and green peppercorns to a boil. Lower to a simmer and set aside.

EXCHANGES
1 CARBOHYDRATE
3 LEAN MEAT

CALORIES 185
 CALORIES FROM FAT 20
TOTAL FAT 2.5 g
 SATURATED FAT 0.6 g
 TRANS FAT 0.0 g
CHOLESTEROL 140 mg
SODIUM 475 mg
POTASSIUM 365 mg
TOTAL CARBOHYDRATE 15 g
 DIETARY FIBER 1 g
 SUGARS 4 g
PROTEIN 28 g
PHOSPHORUS 215 mg

SHASHLIK RUSSIAN-STYLE

SERVES: 6   **SERVING SIZE**: ¹/₆ recipe   **MARINATING TIME**: At least 15 minutes or overnight

I am of Russian descent and this recipe is an authentic version of the large grilled skewers I remember as a child. Pomegranate molasses can be found in many specialty stores. You only need a small amount for a tart fruity flavor. If you like, the meat can be skewered with chunks of onions and peppers.

1 cup plain, fat-free Greek yogurt

¹/₄ cup canola oil

2 tablespoons pomegranate molasses

1 large onion, sliced

3 cloves garlic, minced

1 tablespoon black pepper, ground coarsely

2 pounds lamb cut from the leg in 2-inch cubes (or 2 pounds beef, pork, or chicken, cut in 2-inch cubes)

1. Combine Greek yogurt, oil, pomegranate molasses, onion, garlic, and black pepper in a medium bowl. Pour into a large, tightly sealed plastic bag. Marinate at least 15 minutes at room temperature or overnight in the refrigerator for best results.

2. Preheat grill to medium-high heat and place on grill grate. Cook as per directions for direct heat method (page 3), keeping in mind that 5–8 minutes per side should be enough to cook them through to a medium doneness.

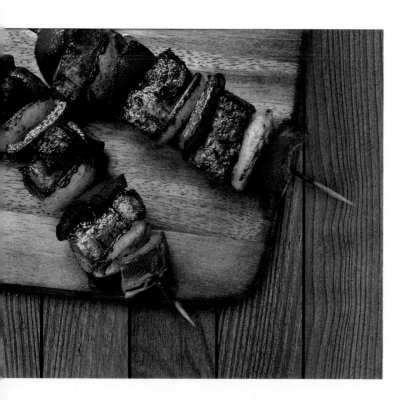

EXCHANGES
5 LEAN MEAT
1 FAT

CALORIES 270
  CALORIES FROM FAT 115
TOTAL FAT 13.0 g
  SATURATED FAT 3.2 g
  TRANS FAT 0.0 g
CHOLESTEROL 100 mg
SODIUM 90 mg
POTASSIUM 470 mg
TOTAL CARBOHYDRATE 5 g
  DIETARY FIBER 0 g
  SUGARS 3 g
PROTEIN 33 g
PHOSPHORUS 280 mg

SPICY PORK TENDERLOINS WITH CHILI AND BLACK VINEGAR

SERVES: 6   **SERVING SIZE**: ¹/₆ recipe   **MARINATING TIME**: At least 15 minutes or overnight

Pork tenders are a totally underappreciated source of protein. They're lean, flavorful, easy to cook, and when marinated, take on flavor very well. One tender will feed 2 people. I often split the tender open and pound it out lightly to form a large ½-inch-thick circle of deliciousness.

¹/₈ cup reduced-sodium soy sauce
 1 tablespoon sesame oil, dark roast
 2 tablespoons Chinese black vinegar or rice vinegar
 1 tablespoon light brown sugar
 1 fresh chili pepper, such as serrano, jalapeño, or Thai bird peppers, seeded and minced
 2 cloves garlic, minced
 1 tablespoon ginger root, minced
 2 pounds pork tenderloins, trimmed of fat

1. Combine soy sauce, sesame oil, vinegar, brown sugar, pepper, garlic, and ginger root in a medium bowl and put into a large, tightly sealed plastic bag. Marinate at least 15 minutes at room temperature or overnight in the refrigerator for best results.

2. Preheat grill to medium-high heat and place on grill grate. Cook as per directions for direct heat method (page 3) for 15–18 minutes, turning occasionally until cooked through and crusted on the outside.

EXCHANGES
4 LEAN MEAT

CALORIES 175
 CALORIES FROM FAT 45
TOTAL FAT 5.0 g
 SATURATED FAT 1.5 g
 TRANS FAT 0.0 g
CHOLESTEROL 80 mg
SODIUM 145 mg
POTASSIUM 480 mg
TOTAL CARBOHYDRATE 2 g
 DIETARY FIBER 0 g
 SUGARS 1 g
PROTEIN 29 g
PHOSPHORUS 265 mg

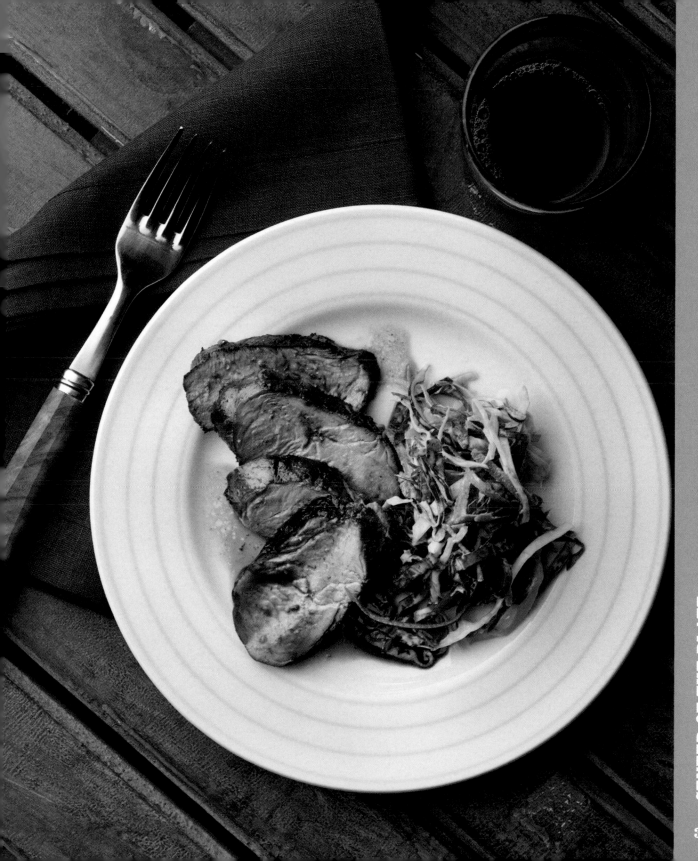

VERACRUZ SNAPPER WITH ORANGE, CAPERS, OLIVES, AND TOMATOES

SERVES: 4   **SERVING SIZE**: ¼ recipe   **MARINATING TIME**: 5 minutes

This is a dish full of warmth, sunshine, and the flavors of Mexico and the Mediterranean. Using a whole, small snapper is traditional, but you can use mahi mahi, grouper, or cod as well. You'll need a fish pan or vegetable pan for the grill if using filets, as they are delicate and can fall apart.

4 filets of snapper (6 ounces each)
1 tablespoon olive oil
   Juice of 1 lime
¼ teaspoon kosher salt
⅛ teaspoon crushed red chili flakes

SAUCE
1 tablespoon olive oil
½ onion, chopped
2 cloves garlic, minced
1 serrano or jalapeño pepper, seeded and minced
3 fresh tomatoes, chopped, or 2 cups canned plum tomatoes, chopped
¼ cup orange juice
¼ cup green olives, chopped
2 tablespoons capers
¼ cup fresh parsley, minced

1. Marinate the snapper together with the oil, lime, salt, and red chili flakes for 5 minutes.

2. Preheat grill to medium-high heat and place on grill grate. Cook as per directions for direct heat method (page 3) for 5–7 minutes, turning the filets once until cooked through and lightly crusted on the outside. Set aside while you make the sauce.

3. Heat the oil over medium-high heat. Sauté the onion, garlic, and chili for 1 minute. Add the tomatoes and orange juice and simmer for 20 minutes until the sauce begins to reduce.

4. Add the olives, capers, and parsley.

EXCHANGES
2 VEGETABLE
5 LEAN MEAT

CALORIES 280
  CALORIES FROM FAT 100
TOTAL FAT 11.0 g
  SATURATED FAT 1.6 g
  TRANS FAT 0.0 g
CHOLESTEROL 60 mg
SODIUM 460 mg
POTASSIUM 1010 mg
TOTAL CARBOHYDRATE 9 g
  DIETARY FIBER 02 g
  SUGARS 5 g
PROTEIN 36 g
PHOSPHORUS 305 mg

GRILLED CHICKEN PICCATA WITH CAPERS, PEARL ONION AND ROAST PEPPER

SERVES: 4   **SERVING SIZE**: ¼ recipe

A total twist on the traditional pan-seared version with a pleasing smoky taste, coupled with sweet roasted peppers and a touch of mellow rich butter.

- 1 tablespoon chopped fresh basil, oregano, or thyme
- 1 teaspoon ground black pepper
- 1 tablespoon olive oil
  Juice of ½ lemon
- 4 (6 ounce) chicken breasts, boneless and skinless, pounded lightly into cutlets
- 2 teaspoons zero–trans-fat, nonhydrogenated buttery spread (such as Smart Balance)
- ¼ cup dry white wine
- 2 tablespoons capers, drained and rinsed
  Juice of 1 lemon
- ½ cup frozen or jarred pearl onions
- ¼ cup roasted red pepper, chopped
- 2 tablespoons fresh chopped, flat leaf parsley

1. Combine chopped fresh herbs, black pepper, olive oil, and lemon juice. Marinate breasts on a shallow dinner plate or large piece of parchment paper.

2. Grill chicken breasts either over coals, gas grill, or in oven (see tips on page 3).

3. In the meantime, heat butter in a large pan over medium-high heat. Add the wine to the pan and simmer, scraping up the bits on the bottom of the pan. Add the capers, lemon juice, pearl onions, and red pepper. Sauté for 1 minute longer and place the grilled chicken back into the pan to swirl into the pan sauce.

4. Sprinkle with chopped parsley and serve.

EXCHANGES
1 VEGETABLE
5 LEAN MEAT

CALORIES 260
 CALORIES FROM FAT 80
TOTAL FAT 9.0 g
 SATURATED FAT 2.1 g
 TRANS FAT 0.0 g
CHOLESTEROL 100 mg
SODIUM 255 mg
POTASSIUM 385 mg
TOTAL CARBOHYDRATE 5 g
 DIETARY FIBER 1 g
 SUGARS 2 g
PROTEIN 37 g
PHOSPHORUS 275 mg

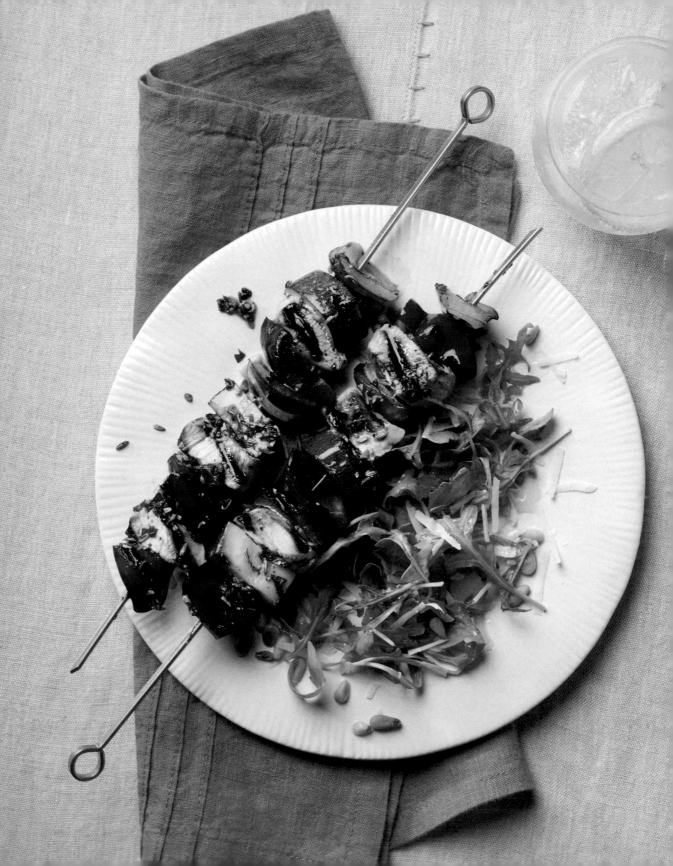

TUSCAN SPIEDINI WITH FRESH HERBS, LEMON, AND CRACKED FENNEL SEEDS

SERVES: 4 **SERVING SIZE:** ¼ recipe **MARINATING TIME:** At least 15 minutes or overnight

Classic in flavor and simplicity, these chicken sticks are wonderful served over orzo pasta, risotto, or a salad. I love them over an arugula salad sprinkled with Parmesan cheese. Fennel seeds give the chicken a very aromatic quality and sweet flavor.

2 tablespoons extra virgin olive oil
 Juice of 1 lemon
2 cloves garlic, minced
2 teaspoons fennel seeds, crushed
½ teaspoon crushed red chili flakes
1 tablespoon fresh oregano, minced
1 tablespoon balsamic vinegar
1 pound boneless skinless chicken breast, cut into 1-inch cubes

1. Combine oil, lemon juice, garlic, fennel seeds, red chili flakes, oregano, and vinegar in a medium bowl and put into a large tightly sealed plastic bag. Marinate at least 15 minutes room temperature or overnight in the refrigerator for best results.

2. Thread the chicken cubes on skewers, either alone or with chunks of your favorite vegetables such as red onion, bell pepper, or zucchini.

3. Preheat grill to medium-high heat and place on grill grate. Cook as per directions for direct heat method (page 3) for 10–12 minutes, turning occasionally, until cooked through and crusted on the outside.

EXCHANGES
4 LEAN MEAT

CALORIES 165
 CALORIES FROM FAT 55
TOTAL FAT 6.0 g
 SATURATED FAT 1.3 g
 TRANS FAT 0.0 g
CHOLESTEROL 65 mg
SODIUM 60 mg
POTASSIUM 220 mg
TOTAL CARBOHYDRATE 1 g
 DIETARY FIBER 0 g
 SUGARS 0 g
PROTEIN 24 g
PHOSPHORUS 180 mg

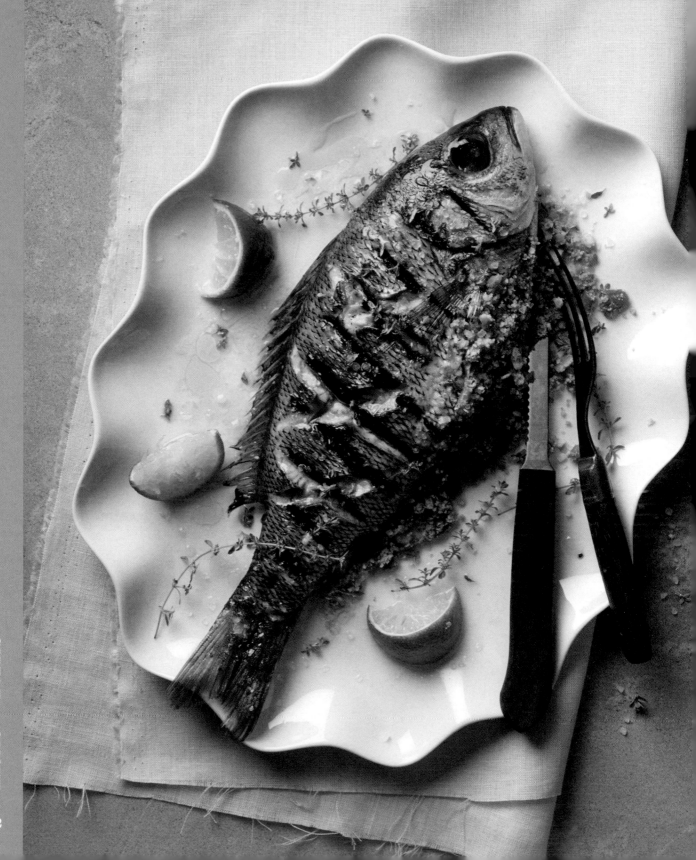

JAMAICAN STUFFED FISH WITH RITZ

SERVES: 4 **SERVING SIZE**: 1/4 recipe

This recipe is a family favorite. The whole fish, normally yellowtail snapper or parrotfish, is stuffed whole, tied with strands of banana leaf, and placed on huge sticks where it is cooked over an open fire.

- 2 small whole fish, such as snapper or trout, cleaned, scaled, and scored in a crisscross pattern
- 1 tablespoon olive oil
  Juice of 1 lime
  Kosher salt, to taste
- 2 cups whole-wheat reduced-fat crackers, crushed
- 1 teaspoon fresh thyme, minced
- 1 hot chili, seeded and minced, such as a Scotch bonnet, serrano, or jalapeño
- 1 bunch scallions, chopped
- 1 tablespoon trans fat–free nonhydrogenated buttery spread (such as Smart Balance), melted
  Toothpicks for securing fish

1. Rub the scored surface of the fish with oil, lime, and salt.

2. Make the stuffing by combining the crushed crackers, thyme, hot chili, scallions, and melted butter in a medium bowl. Fill the cavity of the fish with the stuffing, and using a toothpick or metal skewer, secure the opening by weaving skewer to close fish. You can also stick toothpicks into the bottom of the fish at 2-inch intervals to secure.

3. Preheat grill to medium-high heat and place on grill grate. Cook as per directions for direct heat method (page 3) for 15–18 minutes, turning occasionally, until cooked through and crusted on the outside.

EXCHANGES
2 STARCH
3 LEAN MEAT
1 FAT

CALORIES 335
  CALORIES FROM FAT 110
TOTAL FAT 12.0 g
  SATURATED FAT 2.1 g
  TRANS FAT 0.0 g
CHOLESTEROL 40 mg
SODIUM 370 mg
POTASSIUM 650 mg
TOTAL CARBOHYDRATE 31 g
  DIETARY FIBER 5 g
  SUGARS 6 g
PROTEIN 25 g
PHOSPHORUS 320 mg

CENTER OF THE PLATE

GRILLED CHICKEN SALAD WITH CANDIED PECANS WITH TRIPLE CITRUS VINAIGRETTE

SERVES: 8　**SERVING SIZE**: 1/8 recipe

Sometimes I just crave a simple field green salad with the crunch of nuts, tang of dried fruit, and some simple grilled chicken over the top. This is it.

Olive oil cooking spray
1/4 cup chopped pecans
1 teaspoon sugar
1/8 teaspoon ground red pepper
10 cups fresh salad greens
3/4 cup Triple Citrus Vinaigrette (recipe below)
2 navel oranges, peeled and sectioned
1/4 cup sweetened dried cranberries or apricots (such as Craisins)
2 pounds grilled chicken breast

1. Heat a small nonstick skillet coated with cooking spray over medium-low heat. Add pecans and cook 3–4 minutes or until lightly toasted, stirring frequently. Sprinkle with sugar and red pepper, and cook for 1 minute, stirring constantly. Remove pecans from skillet. Cool on wax paper.

2. Combine greens, Citrus Vinaigrette, and orange sections in a large bowl. Toss well. Place 1 cup greens mixture on each of 8 plates. Top each serving with 1 1/2 teaspoons pecans and 1 1/2 teaspoons cranberries.

3. Top with grilled chicken breast and serve immediately.

TRIPLE CITRUS VINAIGRETTE

SERVES: 16　**SERVING SIZE**: 1 tablespoon

Perfect for summer salads, marinated vegetables, or any protein.

1/4 cup orange juice fresh-squeezed
1/3 cup fresh grapefruit juice
2 tablespoons fresh lemon juice
1 tablespoon extra virgin olive oil
1 tablespoon honey
1 tablespoon Dijon mustard
1 tablespoon low-sodium soy sauce
2 teaspoons minced peeled fresh ginger

1. Combine all ingredients in a blender and process until smooth. Pour into a bowl, cover, and chill.

2. Store in an airtight container in the refrigerator for up to one week.

FOR CHICKEN SALAD WITH VINAIGRETTE	FOR TRIPLE CITRUS VINAIGRETTE ONLY
EXCHANGES	
1 FRUIT	
5 LEAN MEAT	EXCHANGES
	FREE FOOD
CALORIES 275	CALORIES 20
CALORIES FROM FAT 70	CALORIES FROM FAT 10
TOTAL FAT 8.0 g	TOTAL FAT 1.0 g
SATURATED FAT 1.6 g	SATURATED FAT 0.1 g
TRANS FAT 0.0 g	TRANS FAT 0.0 g
CHOLESTEROL 95 mg	CHOLESTEROL 0 mg
SODIUM 185 mg	SODIUM 55 mg
POTASSIUM 520 mg	POTASSIUM 25 mg
TOTAL CARBOHYDRATE 14 g	TOTAL CARBOHYDRATE 2 g
DIETARY FIBER 2 g	DIETARY FIBER 0 g
SUGARS 9 g	SUGARS 2 g
PROTEIN 37 g	PROTEIN 0 g
PHOSPHORUS 295 mg	PHOSPHORUS 0 mg

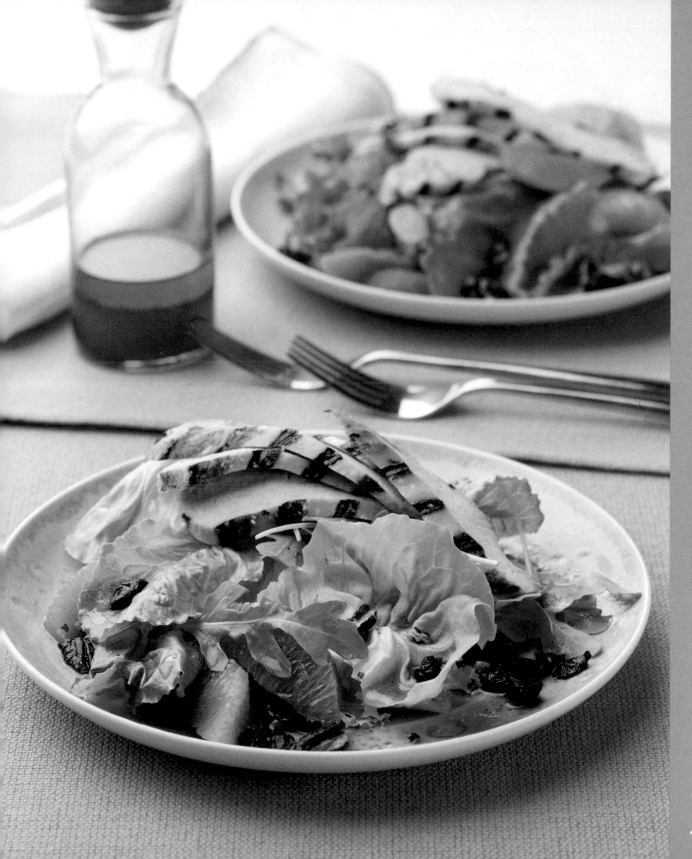

SUNSHINE MOJO CHICKEN

SERVES: 4 **SERVING SIZE**: ¼ recipe **MARINATING TIME:** At least 1 hour or overnight

Every home cook has their own family recipe for mojo (see Chef Steve's Tip). You may use the recipe for Black Coffee Mojo Marinade (page 17) if you prefer. I love them both. Sour orange juice can be found in the ethnic section of most supermarkets. If you can't find it, fresh regular orange juice works, too. If you have the time, marinate the chicken overnight in the refrigerator.

½ cup sour orange juice
1 tablespoon olive oil
1 tablespoon fresh lime juice
2 garlic cloves, minced
1 teaspoon smoked paprika
1 teaspoon dried oregano
½ teaspoon crushed red chili flakes
4 bone-in chicken breast halves, skinned
Cooking spray

1. Combine all the marinade ingredients (through chili flakes) in a large zip-top plastic bag. Add chicken; seal and marinate in refrigerator at least 1 hour or overnight. Drain and discard marinade.

2. Grill chicken as per our recommendations (page 21) until cooked through.

> **CHEF STEVE'S TIP**
> *A mojo, or marinade, is a closely held family recipe that is seldom shared and used often for many things, such as marinating poultry, beef, or pork. Most mojo recipes are generations old.*

EXCHANGES
4 LEAN MEAT

CALORIES 165
  CALORIES FROM FAT 45
TOTAL FAT 5.0 g
  SATURATED FAT 1.1 g
  TRANS FAT 0.0 g
CHOLESTEROL 75 mg
SODIUM 65 mg
POTASSIUM 260 mg
TOTAL CARBOHYDRATE 2 g
  DIETARY FIBER 0 g
  SUGARS 1 g
PROTEIN 27 g
PHOSPHORUS 200 mg

SPLENDID BLENDED MUSHROOM BURGER

SERVES: 6   **SERVING SIZE**: 1 burger

There is something very special about ground beef combined with mushrooms. It is a perfect partnership of flavor and health between the buns.

1 pound lean ground beef

¹/₂ pound shiitake or portabello mushrooms, chopped in a food processor or ground

¹/₂ cup onion, chopped

1 tablespoon steak sauce

1 tablespoon tomato paste

¹/₂ teaspoon black pepper, ground

¹/₂ teaspoon kosher or sea salt

1. In a large mixing bowl, combine all ingredients well and form into 6 burgers by hand.

2. Preheat grill to medium high. Cook as per directions for direct heat method (page 3) for 8–10 minutes, turning once until cooked through and crusted on the outside, while cooked to medium doneness on the inside.

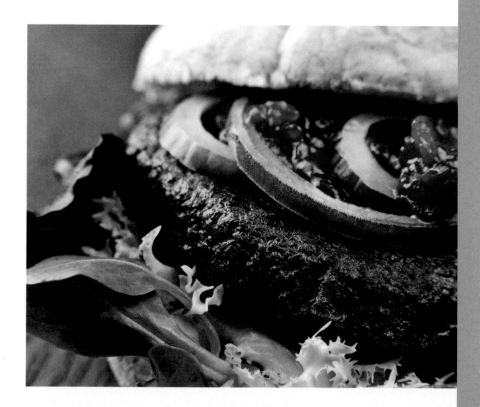

EXCHANGES
1 VEGETABLE
2 LEAN MEAT
¹/₂ FAT

CALORIES 140
  CALORIES FROM FAT 55
TOTAL FAT 6.0 g
  SATURATED FAT 2.5 g
  TRANS FAT 0.4 g
CHOLESTEROL 45 mg
SODIUM 275 mg
POTASSIUM 310 mg
TOTAL CARBOHYDRATE 6 g
  DIETARY FIBER 1 g
  SUGARS 2 g
PROTEIN 15 g
PHOSPHORUS 140 mg

PERSIAN GROUND LAMB STICKS WITH SUMAC

SERVES: 4 **SERVING SIZE**: 2 skewers

My roommate in college was from Iran and was an incredible cook. He taught me how to make these lamb sticks, among many other brilliant recipes. Feel free to use beef if you prefer, although lamb is authentic and goes well with sumac. Sumac is a spice made from dried berries and is red in color and pleasantly tart. It's used in Persian and Middle Eastern cuisines. You can find sumac online or in Middle Eastern grocery stores.

- 1 pound lean ground lamb
- ½ cup onion, chopped
- ½ cup fresh parsley, minced
- 2 cloves garlic, minced
- ½ teaspoon crushed red chili flakes
- ½ teaspoon turmeric
- 2 teaspoons sumac
- 8 wooden or metal skewers

1. In a large bowl, combine all ingredients well.

2. Divide the mixture into 8 parts and form them by hand around the skewers, leaving 2 inches on the bottom to handle.

3. Preheat grill to medium high. Cook as per directions for direct heat method (page 3) for 8–10 minutes, turning once until cooked through and crusted on the outside while remaining cooked to medium on the inside.

EXCHANGES
4 LEAN MEAT

CALORIES 170
 CALORIES FROM FAT 55
TOTAL FAT 6.0 g
 SATURATED FAT 2.2 g
 TRANS FAT 0.0 g
CHOLESTEROL 75 mg
SODIUM 70 mg
POTASSIUM 360 mg
TOTAL CARBOHYDRATE 4 g
 DIETARY FIBER 1 g
 SUGARS 1 g
PROTEIN 24 g
PHOSPHORUS 195 mg

POMEGRANATE LAMB LOLLIPOP CHOPS

SERVES: 4   **SERVING SIZE:** ¼ recipe   **MARINATING TIME:** At least 15 minutes or overnight

I make these for family gatherings and special occasions and am always asked for the recipe. The pomegranate molasses is strong in flavor and you only need a bit to add tart, mouthwatering flavor to any protein. I also grill tofu with the same recipe when cooking meatless. You may use any chop or steak for this recipe as well.

1½ pounds lamb rib chops, trimmed of excess fat
2 tablespoons pomegranate molasses
¼ cup dry red wine
¼ cup fresh mint, chopped
2 garlic cloves, minced
½ onion, sliced
1 teaspoon coarsely ground black pepper

1. Combine all of the marinade ingredients in a medium bowl and put into a large tightly sealed plastic bag. Marinate at least 15 minutes at room temperature or overnight in the refrigerator for best results.

2. Preheat grill to medium high and place on grill grate. Cook as per directions for direct heat method (page 3), keeping in mind that 5–6 minutes per side should be enough to cook the chops through to a medium doneness.

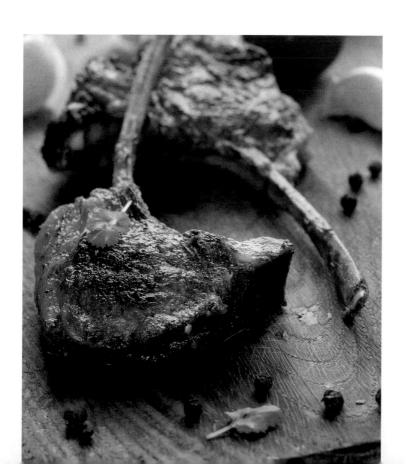

EXCHANGES
3 LEAN MEAT·
½ FAT

CALORIES 175
 CALORIES FROM FAT 65
TOTAL FAT 7.0 g
 SATURATED FAT 2.5 g
 TRANS FAT 0.0 g
CHOLESTEROL 70 mg
SODIUM 60 mg
POTASSIUM 370 mg
TOTAL CARBOHYDRATE 4 g
 DIETARY FIBER 0 g
 SUGARS 2 g
PROTEIN 22 g
PHOSPHORUS 170 mg

GRILLED ZUCCHINI LASAGNA

SERVES: 9   **SERVING SIZE**: 3 × 3-inch square   **MARINATING TIME**: 15 minutes

I make this without pasta. You can incorporate some cooked lasagna noodles if you prefer, or you can add cooked beef, sausage, or crumbled tofu if you like. You may also add grilled slices of eggplant, pepper, onion, or tomatoes. If you bake it the day before serving, it will set up and be easy to cut into squares.

3 medium zucchini, thinly sliced lengthwise
1 tablespoon olive oil
1 tablespoon Italian herb mix, dried
1/2 teaspoon sea or kosher salt
8 ounces fat-free ricotta cheese
1/4 cup egg substitute
1/2 cup Asiago cheese
28 ounces lower-sodium marinara sauce
1 cup fresh basil, chopped
1 cup part-skim mozzarella cheese

1. Marinate zucchini for 15 minutes with olive oil, Italian herbs, and salt.

2. Preheat grill to medium high and place on grill grate. Cook as per directions for direct heat method (page 3), keeping in mind that 3–4 minutes per side should be enough to cook the zucchini through. Do not overcook, as it should be al dente. This step can be done up to 2 days prior to assembling zucchini. Set aside.

3. Preheat oven to 375°F. Spray vegetable oil in a 9 × 9-inch ovenproof baking pan.

4. In a medium mixing bowl, combine ricotta, egg, and Asiago. Set aside.

5. Spoon a little marinara sauce on the bottom of the pan. Arrange a single layer of the zucchini to cover the bottom of the pan.

6. Divide the ricotta mixture in half and spread over the zucchini. Top with more sauce. Sprinkle fresh basil over and top with half the mozzarella. Repeat the process and top with a sprinkle of breadcrumbs, if desired.

7. Bake, covered, for 20 minutes. Remove cover and continue to bake for 10 additional minutes until surface is browned and bubbly.

EXCHANGES
2 VEGETABLE
1 MEDIUM FAT MEAT
1/2 FAT

CALORIES 145
  CALORIES FROM FAT 70
TOTAL FAT 8.0 g
  SATURATED FAT 2.5 g
  TRANS FAT 0.0 g
CHOLESTEROL 20 mg
SODIUM 465 mg
POTASSIUM 495 mg
TOTAL CARBOHYDRATE 10 g
  DIETARY FIBER 2 g
  SUGARS 6 g
PROTEIN 10 g
PHOSPHORUS 180 mg

ESCOVITCH OF TILAPIA WITH SERRANO AND GREEN ONION

SERVES: 4   **SERVING SIZE:** ¼ recipe   **MARINATING TIME:** No more than 10 minutes

This is the Jamaican version of a normally raw marinated dish. My sous chef of many years taught me this recipe. It's typically grilled on foil placed over a wood fire.

1½ pounds white-fleshed fish filets, such as tilapia, snapper, or mahi

2 tablespoons lime juice

2 tablespoons olive oil

1 bunch scallions, chopped

1 tablespoon fresh thyme, minced

⅛ teaspoon ground allspice

1 serrano or jalapeño pepper, seeded and minced

1. In a baking dish or a piece of aluminum foil, marinate the fish filets with all ingredients for no more than 10 minutes or the acid in the lime juice will cook the filets.

2. Preheat grill to medium-high heat. You can cook the filets directly on the foil or place them on a perforated grill grate used for fish or vegetables. Cook as per directions for direct heat method (page 3), keeping in mind that 5–6 minutes per side should be enough to cook them through.

EXCHANGES
4 LEAN MEAT
½ FAT

CALORIES 200
  CALORIES FROM FAT 65
TOTAL FAT 7.0 g
  SATURATED FAT 1.7 g
  TRANS FAT 0.0 g
CHOLESTEROL 75 mg
SODIUM 75 mg
POTASSIUM 530 mg
TOTAL CARBOHYDRATE 1 g
  DIETARY FIBER 0 g
  SUGARS 0 g
PROTEIN 34 g
PHOSPHORUS 265 mg

GRILLED CLAMS WITH GARLIC (BUTTER) AND LIME

SERVES: 4 **SERVING SIZE**: ¼ recipe

I was amazed the first time I made this recipe. Nothing can be easier or more delicious. I prefer the smaller littleneck clams as they are normally sweeter and plump.

2⅔ tablespoons I Can't Believe It's Not Butter
3 cloves garlic, peeled, thinly sliced
½ teaspoon crushed red chili flakes
2 tablespoons parsley, minced
24 littleneck clams, well washed
Juice of 1 lime

1. Melt butter and add the garlic, red chili flakes, and parsley. Place in a small cup and set aside.

2. Preheat grill to high. Place well-washed clams on a piece of foil or cookie baking pan to catch the juices.

3. Cook as per directions for direct heat method (page 3) for 8–10 minutes, turning halfway through, until cooked through and clam shells fully open. Drizzle the butter into the clam shells and serve. Discard any clams that do not open.

EXCHANGES
1 LEAN MEAT
1 FAT

CALORIES 90
  CALORIES FROM FAT 55
TOTAL FAT 6.0 g
  SATURATED FAT 1.4 g
  TRANS FAT 0.0 g
CHOLESTEROL 15 mg
SODIUM 370 mg
POTASSIUM 190 mg
TOTAL CARBOHYDRATE 3 g
  DIETARY FIBER 0 g
  SUGARS 2 g
PROTEIN 7 g
PHOSPHORUS 95 mg

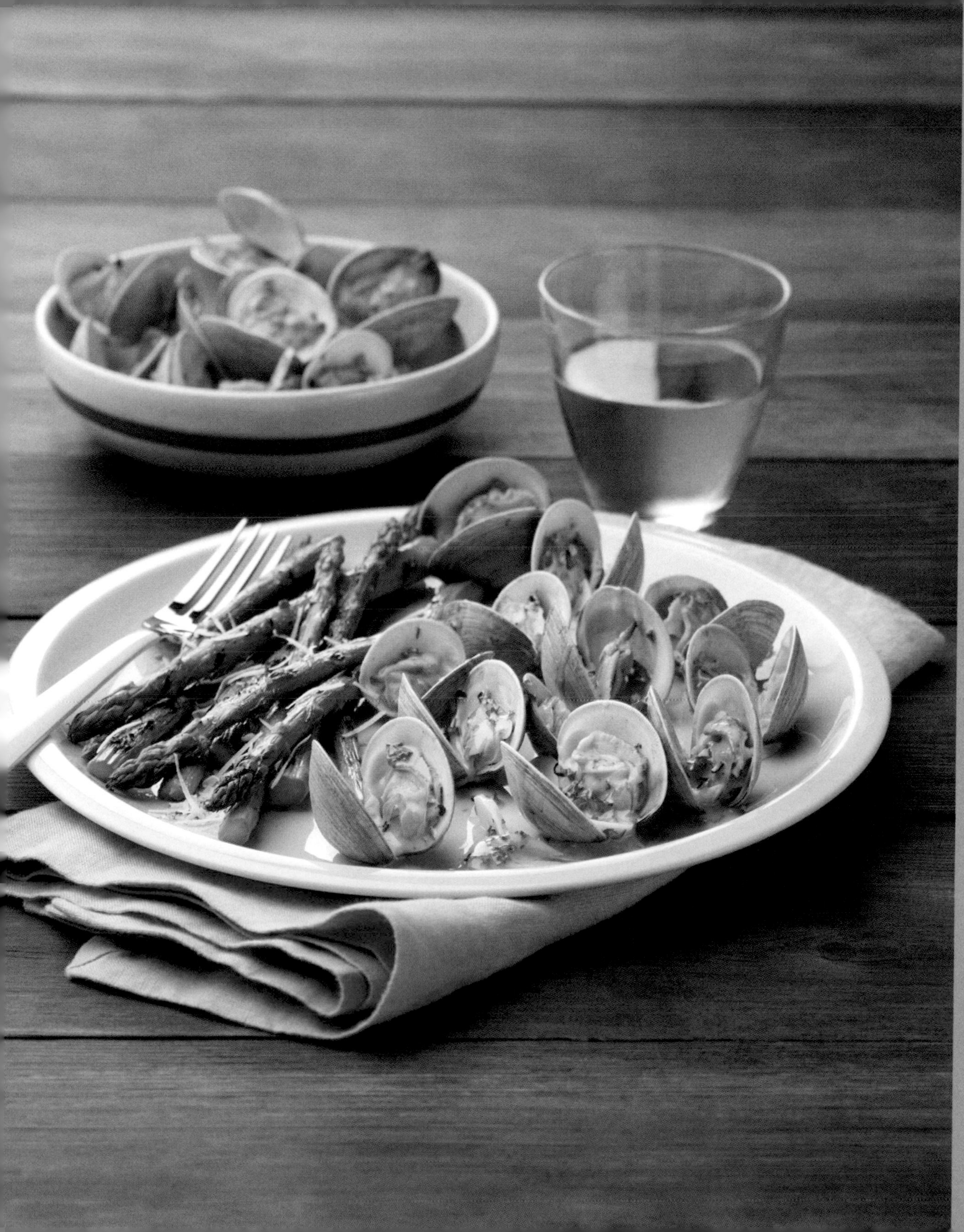

JAPANESE SESAME MISO EGGPLANT STEAKS

SERVES: 4   **SERVING SIZE**: ¼ recipe   **MARINATING TIME**: At least 20 minutes to an hour

I prefer using delicate Japanese eggplants, which have a creamy mild flavor and texture. You can find these long, slender purple beauties in all Asian grocery stores and many produce markets.

4 Japanese eggplants, cut in half lengthwise
½ cup white miso
¼ cup mirin
¼ cup rice vinegar
2 tablespoons low-sodium soy sauce
1 tablespoon sesame oil
1 tablespoon sesame seeds
3 scallions, minced for garnish

1. In a medium mixing bowl, combine the marinade ingredients with a whisk. This can be done up to a few days before grilling. Place the eggplant in a dish large enough to hold it in one layer and pour marinade over. Marinate for at least 20 minutes to an hour.

2. Preheat grill to medium high and place on grill grate. Place the eggplant on the grill cut side down and cook as per directions for direct heat method (page 3) for 4-6 minutes. Turn and repeat process for the other side until eggplants are tender.

3. Garnish with green onions and additional sesame seeds if desired.

EXCHANGES
½ CARBOHYDRATE
3 VEGETABLE
½ FAT

CALORIES 135
  CALORIES FROM FAT 25
TOTAL FAT 3.0 g
  SATURATED FAT 0.4 g
  TRANS FAT 0.0 g
CHOLESTEROL 0 mg
SODIUM 475 mg
POTASSIUM 290 mg
TOTAL CARBOHYDRATE 24 g
  DIETARY FIBER 6 g
  SUGARS 11 g
PROTEIN 3 g
PHOSPHORUS 70 mg

TUNA STEAKS WITH MINT AND GINGER

SERVES: 4   **SERVING SIZE:** 1/4 recipe   **MARINATING TIME:** At least 15 minutes or up to an hour

Elegant and worthy of company, this recipe can also be applied to salmon or swordfish, but when made with tuna, leftover grilled steaks can be sliced thin like Japanese tuna tataki for an incredible appetizer.

MARINADE

- 1 tablespoon extra virgin olive oil
- 1/2 cup orange juice
- Juice of 1 lemon
- 1 tablespoon fresh ginger, minced
- 1/4 cup reduced-sodium soy sauce
- 1 tablespoon fresh mint, minced
- 1/4 teaspoon black pepper, ground coarse

- 4 tuna steaks (6 ounces each), approximately 1 inch thick

1. Combine all of the marinade ingredients in a medium bowl and put into a large, tightly sealed plastic bag. Add tuna steaks and marinate at least 15 minutes at room temperature, or up to an hour in the refrigerator for best results. Discard marinade before cooking.

2. Preheat grill to medium-high heat and place steaks on grill grate. Cook as per directions for direct heat method (page 3), keeping in mind that 3–4 minutes per side should be enough to cook the tuna steaks through to medium doneness.

EXCHANGES
6 LEAN MEAT

CALORIES 285
  CALORIES FROM FAT 90
TOTAL FAT 10.0 g
  SATURATED FAT 2.5 g
  TRANS FAT 0.0 g
CHOLESTEROL 70 mg
SODIUM 345 mg
POTASSIUM 505 mg
TOTAL CARBOHYDRATE 3 g
  DIETARY FIBER 0 g
  SUGARS 2 g
PROTEIN 42 g
PHOSPHORUS 460 mg

MOROCCAN KEFTA

SERVES: 4   **SERVING SIZE**: ¼ recipe

This classic recipe can be made with ground beef, lamb, chicken, or turkey. I love using ground chicken as it is very light and the spice flavors really come through loud and clear. You can form the mixture around skewers or into patties, which are easier to manage. I always serve this dish with couscous or the larger Israeli pearl couscous.

1 pound ground chicken, beef, turkey, or lamb
1 medium red onion, grated
2 cloves garlic, minced
1 teaspoon cumin, ground
½ teaspoon cinnamon, ground
1 teaspoon smoked or regular paprika
1 teaspoon black pepper, ground
2 tablespoons fresh cilantro, minced
1 tablespoon fresh parsley, minced

1. Combine all ingredients well using wet hands, and place the meat mixture in a bowl. Cover, refrigerate, and allow to rest for 20 minutes. You may marinate the meat mixture overnight for better flavor.

2. Form the meat mixture into small patties or around skewers, if preferred.

3. Preheat grill to medium high and place on grill grate. Cook as per directions for direct heat method (page 3), keeping in mind that 3–4 minutes per side should be enough to cook them through to a medium doneness.

EXCHANGES
1 VEGETABLE
3 LEAN MEAT
½ FAT

CALORIES 175
  CALORIES FROM FAT 80
TOTAL FAT 9.0 g
  SATURATED FAT 2.5 g
  TRANS FAT 0.1 g
CHOLESTEROL 85 mg
SODIUM 65 mg
POTASSIUM 635 mg
TOTAL CARBOHYDRATE 5 g
  DIETARY FIBER 1 g
  SUGARS 2 g
PROTEIN 19 g
PHOSPHORUS 205 mg

GRILLED CHICKEN BREAST WITH GRAPEFRUIT POMEGRANATE GLAZE

SERVES: 4   **SERVING SIZE**: ¹/₄ recipe   **MARINATING TIME**: At least 15 minutes or up to an hour

Pomegranate molasses can be found in most Middle Eastern stores and gourmet shops. It's a rich ruby red color with a tart and sweet fruity aftertaste. The grapefruit adds pleasant bitterness to the chicken. After grilling, the chicken is a beautiful mahogany color.

4	chicken breasts (6 ounces each), well trimmed
¹/₄	cup pomegranate molasses
	Juice of 1 grapefruit
1	tablespoon olive oil
¹/₄	cup reduced-sodium soy sauce
1	tablespoon fresh tarragon or basil, minced

1. Combine all of the marinade ingredients in a medium bowl and put into a large tightly sealed plastic bag. Marinate chicken breasts at least 15 minutes at room temperature or up to an hour in the refrigerator for best results.

2. Preheat grill to medium high and place on grill grate. Cook as per directions for direct heat method (page 3), keeping in mind that 5–6 minutes per side should be enough to cook the chicken through to completion. (See Test Chicken for Doneness, page 21.)

CHEF STEVE'S TIP

Many of our recipes call for fresh herbs. When I'm out in the field cooking for restaurants and super markets, I use a combination of dried and fresh herbs. Here's the chef's rule of thumb: Dried herbs are always added at the beginning of a recipe to expand the flavor when sautéed in oil or other fats, while fresh herbs are always added at the end of a cooking process, so the delicate oils stay in your dish.

EXCHANGES
¹/₂ CARBOHYDRATE
5 LEAN MEAT

CALORIES 245
 CALORIES FROM FAT 55
TOTAL FAT 6.0 g
 SATURATED FAT 1.4 g
 TRANS FAT 0.0 g
CHOLESTEROL 100 mg
SODIUM 360 mg
POTASSIUM 490 mg
TOTAL CARBOHYDRATE 8 g
 DIETARY FIBER 0 g
 SUGARS 6 g
PROTEIN 37 g
PHOSPHORUS 280 mg

THAI GRILLED CHICKEN DRUMSTICKS WITH CILANTRO AND LIME

SERVES: 6   **SERVING SIZE:** 1 drumstick   **MARINATING TIME:** At least 15 minutes or overnight

These drumsticks have a spicy little kick and are great when paired with a salad.

MARINADE

- 1 tablespoon peanut or canola oil
- 3 cloves garlic, minced
- 2 stalks lemongrass, trimmed and minced
- ¼ cup fresh cilantro, minced
- 1 tablespoon fresh ginger, minced
- 2 tablespoons fish sauce
- 1 tablespoon dark brown sugar
- 2 serrano, jalapeño, or Scotch bonnet peppers, seeded and minced
  Juice of 2 limes

- 6 chicken legs or boneless, skinless chicken thighs, scored in a crisscross fashion with a sharp knife

1. Combine all of the marinade ingredients in a medium bowl and put into a large, tightly sealed plastic bag. Marinate chicken at least 15 minutes at room temperature or overnight in the refrigerator for best results. Discard marinade before cooking.

2. Preheat grill to medium high and place on grill grate. Cook as per directions for direct heat method (page 3), keeping in mind that 6–8 minutes per side should be enough to cook the chicken through to completion. (See Test Chicken for Doneness, page 21.)

EXCHANGES
2 LEAN MEAT
½ FAT

CALORIES 110
  CALORIES FROM FAT 35
TOTAL FAT 4.0 g
  SATURATED FAT 0.9 g
  TRANS FAT 0.0 g
CHOLESTEROL 45 mg
SODIUM 285 mg
POTASSIUM 175 mg
TOTAL CARBOHYDRATE 3 g
  DIETARY FIBER 0 g
  SUGARS 1 g
PROTEIN 14 g
PHOSPHORUS 100 mg

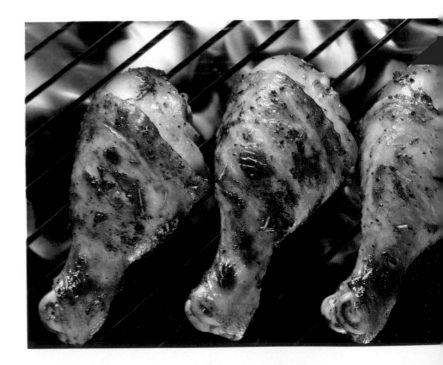

LEMONGRASS BEEF

SERVES: 6   **SERVING SIZE:** 1/6 recipe   **MARINATING TIME:** At least 15 minutes or up to an hour

Once it's grilled, you can enjoy this lemongrass beef as is or make an incredible grilled beef and noodle salad from it. You can use flank steak, skirt steak, or flap meat, also known as tri tips. If you have the time, marinate overnight to make the flavor more pronounced.

MARINADE

- 3 stalks lemongrass, outer husk layer removed, and minced
- 3 cloves garlic, minced
- 2 tablespoons fish sauce
- 1 tablespoon brown sugar
- 2 serrano or Thai chili peppers, seeded and minced
- 1 tablespoon peanut or canola oil
  Juice of 1 lime

1 1/2 pounds skirt or flank steak

1. Combine all of the marinade ingredients in a medium bowl and put into a large tightly sealed plastic bag. Marinate beef at least 15 minutes at room temperature, or overnight in the refrigerator for best results.

2. Preheat grill to medium high and place on grill grate. Cook as per directions for direct heat method (page 3), keeping in mind that 5–6 minutes per side should be enough to cook the beef thoroughly to medium.

EXCHANGES
3 LEAN MEAT
1/2 FAT

CALORIES 170
 CALORIES FROM FAT 65
TOTAL FAT 7.0 g
 SATURATED FAT 2.7 g
 TRANS FAT 0.0 g
CHOLESTEROL 60 mg
SODIUM 280 mg
POTASSIUM 335 mg
TOTAL CARBOHYDRATE 3 g
 DIETARY FIBER 0 g
 SUGARS 1 g
PROTEIN 23 g
PHOSPHORUS 180 mg

VIET SPICED COFFEE CHICKEN SATES

SERVES: 8   **SERVING SIZE**: 3 skewers   **MARINATING TIME**: At least 15 minutes or overnight

Spicy, sweet, and exotic, the flavor of coffee and curry are blended together perfectly by the nutty taste of peanut butter. You may also use a tender cut of beef, lamb, or pork for this marinade. The marinade can be made a day before marinating your favorite protein. If you have the time, marinating the chicken or meat overnight in the refrigerator is the best way to increase flavor.

MARINADE

   1 tablespoon canola or peanut oil
 1/4 cup reduced-sodium soy sauce
   2 tablespoons peanut butter, smooth or chunky
   1 tablespoon curry powder
   2 tablespoons ground coffee
   1 tablespoon light brown sugar
   2 tablespoons lime juice
   3 cloves minced garlic
   1 tablespoon minced fresh ginger root
   1 teaspoon crushed red chilies

   2 pounds boneless, skinless chicken breast cut into 1/2-inch-wide strips
  24 wooden skewers

1. Combine the marinade ingredients in a medium bowl and pour mixture into a large tightly sealed plastic bag with chicken. Marinate at least 15 minutes room temperature or overnight in the refrigerator for best results.

2. Preheat grill to medium high and place chicken on skewers. Arrange skewers on grill grate. Cook as per directions for direct heat method (page 3), keeping in mind that 5–6 minutes per side should be enough to cook them completely through.

EXCHANGES
4 LEAN MEAT

CALORIES 160
  CALORIES FROM FAT 45
TOTAL FAT 5.0 g
  SATURATED FAT 1.1 g
  TRANS FAT 0.0 g
CHOLESTEROL 65 mg
SODIUM 205 mg
POTASSIUM 245 mg
TOTAL CARBOHYDRATE 3 g
  DIETARY FIBER 0 g
  SUGARS 1 g
PROTEIN 25 g
PHOSPHORUS 190 mg

CHIPOTLE CHILI AND TEA RUBBED SALMON

SERVES: 8 **SERVING SIZE:** ⅛ recipe **MARINATING TIME:** 20 minutes

Spice rubs are simple to make in a blender and keep for weeks refrigerated. This rub is a rich, ruby color with deep complex spicy flavors of chili, tea, and lime. It can be made with either dried reconstituted chipotle chili peppers or canned chili peppers in adobo. This rub is wonderful on seafood, meat, poultry, or vegetables. This recipe makes enough spice rub for 2 pounds of salmon or chicken. You may keep the remainder of the spice rub in your refrigerator for future use.

4 chipotle chili peppers in adobo
1 tablespoon olive or canola oil
1 tablespoon light brown sugar
1 tablespoon ground tea leaves, green or black
1 teaspoon oregano
2 teaspoons coarse salt
1 tablespoon lime juice

1 2-pound side of salmon, skin removed

1. Place all the ingredients except salmon in a blender, or use a small hand-held immersion blender and purée ingredients together until smooth.

2. Rub mixture over the surface of the salmon. Place the salmon on a baking dish and marinate for 20 minutes.

3. Preheat grill to medium high. You can cook the salmon directly on a piece of foil or place them on a perforated grill grate used for fish or vegetables. Cook as per directions for direct heat method (page 3), keeping in mind that 5–6 minutes per side should be enough to cook through.

4. Cool for 30 minutes before serving.

EXCHANGES
4 LEAN MEAT
1 FAT

CALORIES 225
CALORIES FROM FAT 110
TOTAL FAT 12.0 g
SATURATED FAT 2.0 g
TRANS FAT 0.0 g
CHOLESTEROL 80 mg
SODIUM 435 mg
POTASSIUM 370 mg
TOTAL CARBOHYDRATE 2 g
DIETARY FIBER 0 g
SUGARS 2 g
PROTEIN 25 g
PHOSPHORUS 255 mg

GRILLED PORTABELLAS WITH TOMATO AND TUSCAN HERBS

SERVES: 6   **SERVING SIZE**: 1 mushroom cap   **MARINATING TIME**: At least 15–30 minutes

I love these 'shrooms as a sandwich topped with a slice of fresh mozzarella or provolone and served on a ciabatta roll or great Italian bread. They are great when served alongside a mixed green salad.

¼ cup extra virgin olive oil

2 tablespoons lemon juice

2 tablespoons balsamic vinegar

1 tablespoon fresh oregano, minced

1 sprig fresh rosemary, minced

2 tablespoons basil, minced

2 cloves garlic, minced

½ cup tomato, chopped

½ teaspoon black pepper

6 portabello mushrooms, wiped clean and stem removed

1. Combine all of the marinade ingredients in a medium bowl and put into a large tightly sealed plastic bag. Marinate mushroom caps at least 15–30 minutes at room temperature for best results.

2. Preheat grill to medium high and place mushroom caps on grill grate. Cook as per directions for direct heat method (page 3), keeping in mind that 5 minutes per side should be enough to cook them completely through to tender. Baste occasionally with additional marinade while cooking. You can pour any leftover marinade over mushrooms before serving.

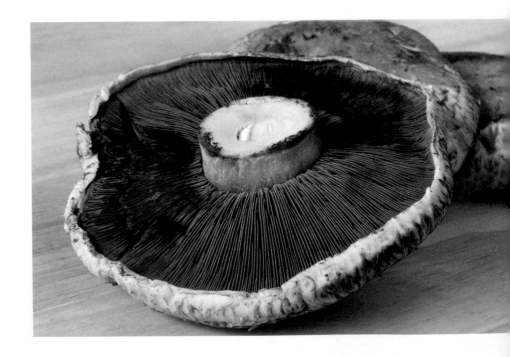

EXCHANGES
1 VEGETABLE
2 FAT

CALORIES 105
  CALORIES FROM FAT 80
TOTAL FAT 9.0 g
  SATURATED FAT 1.3 g
  TRANS FAT 0.0 g
CHOLESTEROL 0 mg
SODIUM 5 mg
POTASSIUM 315 mg
TOTAL CARBOHYDRATE 5 g
  DIETARY FIBER 1 g
  SUGARS 2 g
PROTEIN 2 g
PHOSPHORUS 75 mg

MARGARITA MARINATED SKIRT STEAK

SERVES: 8   SERVING SIZE: ⅛ recipe   **MARINATING TIME:** At least 30 minutes or overnight

You can toast your guests with this wonderful summertime dish, or anytime during the year. Serve it with Romesco Sauce (page 88). Make sure you slice against the grain, so the beef will be tender.

MARINADE

2 tablespoons canola oil
Juice of 2 limes
Juice of 1 orange
¼ cup tequila
2 tablespoons soy sauce
¼ cup cilantro, minced
3 scallions, minced
1 jalapeño, seeded and minced
2 cloves garlic, minced

2 pounds skirt steak or flap meat, trimmed well of excess fat

1. Combine all of the marinade ingredients in a medium bowl and put into a large tightly sealed plastic bag. Marinate beef at least 30 minutes or overnight in the refrigerator for best results.

2. Preheat grill to medium high and place beef on grill grate. Cook as per directions for direct heat method (page 3), keeping in mind that 4–5 minutes per side should be enough to cook the beef through to medium doneness. Baste occasionally with additional marinade while cooking.

EXCHANGES
4 LEAN MEAT
1½ FAT

CALORIES 250
CALORIES FROM FAT 115
TOTAL FAT 13.0 g
SATURATED FAT 3.7 g
TRANS FAT 0.0 g
CHOLESTEROL 75 mg
SODIUM 295 mg
POTASSIUM 345 mg
TOTAL CARBOHYDRATE 3 g
DIETARY FIBER 0 g
SUGARS 2 g
PROTEIN 25 g
PHOSPHORUS 225 mg

GRILLED PIZZA A FEW WAYS

SERVES: 16   **SERVING SIZE**: 1 piece

Pizza is unique and delicious on the grill. You have to have all your topping ingredients ready to roll when the pizza goes on the grill because it cooks up fast. This recipe calls for store-bought pizza dough, but you can make your own if you have the time. Remember, working quickly is key here to a perfectly grilled pizza.

4 small whole-wheat pizza dough balls (about 6 ounces each)
4 teaspoons olive oil for brushing grill
1 cup favorite tomato sauce
1/8 cup chopped olives
1/8 cup sliced red onion
1/8 cup sliced mushrooms
1 1/4 cups part-skim mozzarella cheese, shredded
1/2 cup cooked sliced sausage or pepperoni (optional)
1/4 cup fresh basil, shredded

1. Preheat the grill to medium heat.

2. Use a rolling pin to flatten dough balls to about 1/2 inch thick, or a bit thinner depending on preference.

3. Brush the grill with oil and carefully place one pizza at a time on grill. If you're a grill master, you can do 2 at a time. The dough begins to cook and puff up instantly. When the bottom of the crust turns brown, lightly brush the top side with olive oil and flip the crust over, using a spatula.

4. Divide the tomato sauce evenly among the four pizzas and quickly top the pizzas with tomato sauce. Add as many or as few of the ingredients as you prefer, close the lid, and cook for approximately 2 minutes until the cheese melts. Remove from the grill and repeat the process to cook the other pizzas. Cut each pizza into four slices.

EXCHANGES
1 STARCH
1 FAT

CALORIES 125
 CALORIES FROM FAT 35
TOTAL FAT 4.0 g
 SATURATED FAT 1.2 g
 TRANS FAT 0.0 g
CHOLESTEROL 5 mg
SODIUM 320 mg
POTASSIUM 140 mg
TOTAL CARBOHYDRATE 19 g
 DIETARY FIBER 2 g
 SUGARS 1 g
PROTEIN 5 g
PHOSPHORUS 120 mg

HONEY STONE GROUND MUSTARD CHICKEN

SERVES: 4–6 **SERVING SIZE**: ¹⁄₆ recipe **MARINATING TIME**: At least 30 minutes or overnight

These classic roadhouse chicken breasts taste way better than most restaurants as this sauce is simple and flavorful. They are great on a sandwich as well.

MARINADE

1 tablespoon olive oil

2 tablespoons Dijon-style mustard

2 tablespoons stone-ground mustard

1 tablespoon honey

1 tablespoon lemon juice

2 pounds boneless, skinless chicken breasts, trimmed well

1. Combine all of the marinade ingredients in a medium bowl and put into a large, tightly sealed plastic bag. Marinate chicken breasts at least 30 minutes or overnight in the refrigerator for best results.

2. Preheat grill to medium high and place chicken on grill grate. Cook as per directions for direct heat method (page 3), keeping in mind that 8–10 minutes per side should be enough to cook the chicken through to doneness. (See Test Chicken for Doneness, page 21.)

EXCHANGES
¹⁄₂ CARBOHYDRATE
4 LEAN MEAT

CALORIES 215
 CALORIES FROM FAT 55
TOTAL FAT 6.0 g
 SATURATED FAT 1.4 g
 TRANS FAT 0.0 g
CHOLESTEROL 90 mg
SODIUM 270 mg
POTASSIUM 285 mg
TOTAL CARBOHYDRATE 5 g
 DIETARY FIBER 1 g
 SUGARS 3 g
PROTEIN 32 g
PHOSPHORUS 245 mg

GRILLED HAWAIIAN CHICKEN WITH PINEAPPLE AND CANADIAN BACON

SERVES: 6   **SERVING SIZE:** ¹/₆ recipe   **MARINATING TIME:** At least 30 minutes or overnight

You'll never be able to eat commercial substitutes again after trying this simple recipe. Feel free to make extra marinade to drizzle over chicken after cooking.

2 pounds boneless, skinless chicken breasts or thighs, trimmed of excess fat and pounded lightly

6 slices fresh pineapple, ¹/₂ inch thick

6 slices Canadian bacon

MARINADE

¹/₄ cup low-sodium soy sauce

¹/₂ cup unsweetened pineapple juice

2 tablespoons tomato catsup

1 tablespoon minced fresh ginger

3 scallions minced

1. Combine all of the marinade ingredients in a medium bowl and put into a large, tightly sealed plastic bag. Marinate chicken breasts at least 30 minutes or overnight in the refrigerator for best results.

2. Preheat grill to medium high and place beef on grill grate. Cook as per directions for direct heat method (page 3), keeping in mind that 8–10 minutes per side should be enough to cook the chicken through to doneness. (See Test Chicken for Doneness, page 21.) Set cooked chicken breast aside.

3. Place pineapple and Canadian bacon slices on heated grill for 2 minutes and turn over. Repeat process until marked and then top each cooked chicken breast with a slice of pineapple and bacon before serving.

EXCHANGES
1 FRUIT
5 LEAN MEAT

CALORIES 265
  CALORIES FROM FAT 55
TOTAL FAT 6.0 g
  SATURATED FAT 1.7 g
  TRANS FAT 0.0 g
CHOLESTEROL 100 mg
SODIUM 465 mg
POTASSIUM 485 mg
TOTAL CARBOHYDRATE 13 g
  DIETARY FIBER 1 g
  SUGARS 11 g
PROTEIN 38 g
PHOSPHORUS 315 mg

PORK TENDERLOINS WITH SPICY MAPLE BOURBON GLAZE

SERVES: 6 **SERVING SIZE**: ¹/₆ recipe **MARINATING TIME**: At least 30 minutes or overnight

Pork tenders are one of the most underutilized cuts of meat ever. They are very lean, juicy, flavorful, and absorb any flavors that they are marinated with. The sauce thickens and caramelizes, which calms the heat of the Sriracha sauce.

2 pounds pork tenderloins, trimmed well
1 cup sugar-free cola or ginger ale
1 tablespoon orange zest
2 tablespoons maple syrup
½ cup bourbon
2 tablespoons Sriracha sauce

1. Combine all of the marinade ingredients in a medium bowl and put into a large tightly sealed plastic bag. Marinate at least 30 minutes or overnight in the refrigerator for best results.

2. Remove tenderloins from marinade and drain well. Preheat grill to medium high and place the tenderloins on grill grate. Cook as per directions for indirect heat method (page 3) for 30 minutes, turning halfway through. Baste with marinade for another 15–20 minutes, cooking over moderate heat until pork is cooked through.

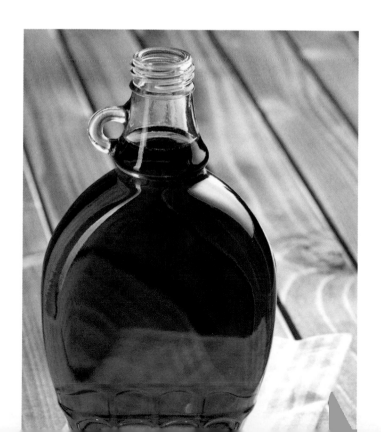

EXCHANGES
¹/₂ CARBOHYDRATE
4 LEAN MEAT

CALORIES 195
  CALORIES FROM FAT 35
TOTAL FAT 4.0 g
  SATURATED FAT 1.3 g
  TRANS FAT 0.0 g
CHOLESTEROL 80 mg
SODIUM 160 mg
POTASSIUM 495 mg
TOTAL CARBOHYDRATE 6 g
  DIETARY FIBER 0 g
  SUGARS 5 g
PROTEIN 30 g
PHOSPHORUS 265 mg

MANHATTAN-SIDEWALK-STYLE GRILLED SAUSAGE AND PEPPERS

SERVES: 8 **SERVING SIZE**: $1/8$ recipe

OK. Yes, I'm a New Yorker and can still smell the aroma of sausage and peppers served from street carts way before street food was popular. My version is lighter and made with much less grease and toil. There are many great sausages now available with a much lower fat percentage made from turkey and chicken.

8 sausages (3 ounces each); you can use pork, chicken, or turkey
2 tablespoons olive oil
1 tablespoon balsamic vinegar
1 red pepper, halved, seeded
1 green pepper, halved, seeded
1 yellow pepper, halved, seeded
2 long hot peppers, left whole
1 red onion, peeled and cut into thick rings
$1/4$ cup basil, shredded
$1/4$ teaspoon salt

1. Preheat grill to medium high and place sausages on grill. Cook as per directions for direct heat method (page 3). Cook for 8–10 minutes until sausages are cooked through and then set aside.

2. In a large bowl, combine olive oil, vinegar, peppers, and onion. Place the vegetables on a grill pan over the grill and cook as per directions for direct heat method (page 3). Cook for 5–6 minutes until lightly browned and tender. Set aside to cool.

3. When vegetables are cool, slice peppers into 1-inch-thick slices, combine with onion, chop long hot peppers, and add basil and season with salt.

4. Slice cooked sausages and combine with grilled peppers. Serve alone, on Italian bread, or over pasta.

EXCHANGES
2 VEGETABLE
2 LEAN MEAT
1$1/2$ FAT

CALORIES 200
 CALORIES FROM FAT 100
TOTAL FAT 11.0 g
 SATURATED FAT 2.5 g
 TRANS FAT 0.0 g
CHOLESTEROL 65 mg
SODIUM 555 mg
POTASSIUM 390 mg
TOTAL CARBOHYDRATE 9 g
 DIETARY FIBER 1 g
 SUGARS 5 g
PROTEIN 16 g
PHOSPHORUS 190 mg

KILLER CANTON TURKEY BURGERS

SERVES: 4   **SERVING SIZE**: 1 burger

Tired of the same old turkey burgers? I was, until I created this recipe.

1 pound lean ground turkey

6 scallions, minced

1 carrot, grated

⅓ cup water chestnuts, chopped

1 tablespoon minced fresh ginger

1 tablespoon reduced-sodium soy sauce

1 tablespoon Hoisin sauce

1 tablespoon sesame oil

2 tablespoons cilantro, minced

1 tablespoon lemongrass, minced (optional)

1. Combine all the ingredients in a large bowl and shape into 4–6 patties.

2. Preheat grill to medium high and place beef on grill grate. Cook as per directions for direct heat method (page 3), keeping in mind that 4–5 minutes per side should be enough to cook the burgers through to doneness. (See Test Chicken for Doneness, page 21.)

EXCHANGES
1 VEGETABLE
3 LEAN MEAT
1½ FAT

CALORIES 240
  CALORIES FROM FAT 115
TOTAL FAT 13.0 g
  SATURATED FAT 3.0 g
  TRANS FAT 0.1 g
CHOLESTEROL 85 mg
SODIUM 295 mg
POTASSIUM 405 mg
TOTAL CARBOHYDRATE 7 g
  DIETARY FIBER 2 g
  SUGARS 3 g
PROTEIN 24 g
PHOSPHORUS 235 mg

BAHN MI SANDWICH

SERVES: 6   **SERVING SIZE**: ¹⁄₆ recipe

Bahn Mi sandwiches are traditional Vietnamese hero sandwiches, which have become quite popular over the last few years. They always contain some kind of grilled meat or tofu, pickled vegetables, fresh cilantro, and fiery raw jalapeño slices. Here they take the form of a burger. I prefer ground chicken or turkey, but beef and lamb also work great. I use simple tofu planks for this recipe.

1 24-inch French baguette, cut in half lengthwise
1 pound tofu, sliced in ¹⁄₂-inch-thick slices from the short side
2 tablespoons reduced-sodium soy sauce or fish sauce
1 tablespoon sesame oil

PICKLED VEGETABLES
1 cup carrot, cut in matchsticks
¹⁄₃ cup rice or white vinegar
2 teaspoons agave or ¹⁄₂ teaspoon Splenda

SPICY MAYONNAISE
¹⁄₂ cup low-fat mayonnaise
1 tablespoon Sriracha

1 jalapeño, thinly sliced
¹⁄₂ bunch cilantro sprigs

1. Heat French baguette in 325°F oven until warm.

2. Marinate the tofu in soy sauce and sesame oil at least 20 minutes at room temperature or overnight in the refrigerator.

3. Place all the Pickled Vegetables ingredients in a small saucepan. Bring to a boil and pour into a bowl to cool. This can be done up to 3 days before assembling.

4. In a small bowl, mix together mayonnaise and Sriracha. This can be done up to 3 days before assembly.

5. Preheat grill to medium high and place tofu on grill grate. Cook as per directions for direct heat method (page 3), keeping in mind that 4–5 minutes per side should be enough to mark the tofu and color it golden brown. Set aside.

6. Spread the entire baguette with spicy mayo. Layer the tofu over the mayo. Arrange the pickled vegetables over tofu. Scatter the jalapeño and cilantro on top. Cover with baguette.

7. Cut sandwich into 2-inch-wide wedges and serve.

EXCHANGES
2 STARCH
1 CARBOHYDRATE
1 MEDIUM FAT MEAT

CALORIES 290
  CALORIES FROM FAT 70
TOTAL FAT 8.0 g
  SATURATED FAT 1.5 g
  TRANS FAT 0.0 g
CHOLESTEROL 0 mg
SODIUM 580 mg
POTASSIUM 330 mg
TOTAL CARBOHYDRATE 43 g
  DIETARY FIBER 3 g
  SUGARS 7 g
PROTEIN 14 g
PHOSPHORUS 180 mg

SPICY SPANISH STYLE SHRIMP AND SCALLOP SKEWERS

SERVES: 6   **SERVING SIZE**: 1 skewer   **MARINATING TIME**: 30 minutes

These skewers are so easy to make and so loaded with authentic Spanish taste. I offer the option of including leftover cooked sausage on these skewers, which is how I remember having them on my last trip to the Andalusian region of Spain. If using wooden skewers, soak them in water for at least 30 minutes, so they don't burn on the grill.

1 pound large shrimp, peeled and deveined
1 pound medium scallops
2 tablespoons extra virgin olive oil
2 cloves garlic, minced
2 teaspoons smoked paprika
$\frac{1}{2}$ teaspoon crushed red chili flakes
1 teaspoon oregano
  Juice of 1 lemon
2 tablespoons parsley, chopped
2 cooked sausages, cut into 1-inch-thick slices
  (optional)
6 metal or soaked wooden skewers

1. Combine all of the marinade ingredients in a medium bowl and put into a large tightly sealed plastic bag. Marinate 30 minutes in the refrigerator for best results.

2. Place the shrimp and scallops alternately on skewers. If using the cooked sausage, thread them on as well.

3. Preheat grill to medium high and place skewers on grill grate. Cook as per directions for direct heat method (page 3), keeping in mind that 4–5 minutes per side should be enough to cook the shellfish through to doneness. They should be totally opaque once cooked through.

EXCHANGES
$\frac{1}{2}$ CARBOHYDRATE
3 LEAN MEAT

CALORIES 175
  CALORIES FROM FAT 45
TOTAL FAT 5.0 g
  SATURATED FAT 0.8 g
  TRANS FAT 0.0 g
CHOLESTEROL 150 mg
SODIUM 455 mg
POTASSIUM 390 mg
TOTAL CARBOHYDRATE 5 g
  DIETARY FIBER 0 g
  SUGARS 0 g
PROTEIN 28 g
PHOSPHORUS 405 mg

AZTEC TURKEY QUINOA BURGERS

SERVES: 6 **SERVING SIZE**: 1 burger

Yumburgers, that's what I call them. Try serving them with avocado and the pickled vegetables from the Bahn Mi Sandwich (page 70). Come to think of it, the Spicy Mayonnaise is also incredible on these burgers.

1 pound lean ground turkey or chicken

1/3 cup cooked quinoa, golden or red

3 scallions, minced

1/2 cup kale, chopped

2 tablespoons extra virgin olive oil

1/2 teaspoon cumin

1 teaspoon oregano

1 teaspoon chili powder

1 chipotle chili en adobo, minced (optional)

1. In a large bowl, combine all ingredients and mix well to distribute. Shape into 6 patties.

2. Preheat grill to medium high and place burgers on grill grate. Cook as per directions for direct heat method (page 3), keeping in mind that 5–6 minutes per side should be enough to cook the burgers through to doneness. (See Test Chicken for Doneness, page 21.)

EXCHANGES
2 LEAN MEAT

CALORIES 175
 CALORIES FROM FAT 100
TOTAL FAT 11.0 g
 SATURATED FAT 2.3 g
 TRANS FAT 0.1 g
CHOLESTEROL 55 mg
SODIUM 60 mg
POTASSIUM 245 mg
TOTAL CARBOHYDRATE
 4 g
 DIETARY FIBER 1 g
 SUGARS 1 g
PROTEIN 16 g
PHOSPHORUS 170 mg

HARISSA MARINATED CHICKEN LEGS

SERVES: 6   **SERVING SIZE:** 1 chicken leg

You may use any dried chili for this recipe; many supermarkets carry these in the Latin food section. I recommend the Harissa (see Chef Steve's Tip). If you can't find them, use canned chipotle chili en adobo.

5 dried arbol chilis
5 dried Anaheim or New Mexico chilis
1 teaspoon caraway seeds
1 teaspoon cumin seeds
1 teaspoon coriander seeds
3 cloves garlic
¼ cup olive oil
6 large bone-in chicken legs

CHEF STEVE'S TIP

Harissa is a North African fiery spice paste that I first sampled in Morocco. It's made with dried chili and an assortment of spices. I keep a jar in my fridge, as it stays for 2 weeks and it can be used as a spice rub, sauce, or mixed into cooked rice, couscous, pasta and even whipped into cooked potatoes. You will have more Harissa than you need—go ahead and save the extra for the next time you make this favorite recipe.

EXCHANGES
3 LEAN MEAT
1 FAT

CALORIES 185
  CALORIES FROM FAT 100
TOTAL FAT 11.0 g
  SATURATED FAT 2.4 g
  TRANS FAT 0.0 g
CHOLESTEROL 105 mg
SODIUM 70 mg
POTASSIUM 360 mg
TOTAL CARBOHYDRATE 2 g
  DIETARY FIBER 1 g
  SUGARS 1 g
PROTEIN 19 g
PHOSPHORUS 170 mg

1. Remove the stems and seeds from the dried chili peppers and place them in a heatproof bowl. Boil some water and pour over chilis. Allow them to sit in the hot water for about 45 minutes, drain and squeeze out the excess moisture. Save ¼ cup of the water.

2. While the chilis are soaking, heat a small sauté pan over medium heat and toast all the dried seeds until you can smell the fragrance released by the toasting seeds. Grind the seeds in a coffee bean grinder.

3. Place the chilis, seeds, and garlic in a food processor or blender fitted with a standard S blade and puree, slowly adding the oil and some of the reserved water until a smooth paste is formed.

4. Score 6 large bone-in chicken legs in a crisscross fashion using a paring or French knife.

5. Combine chicken legs and 1 cup of the Harissa in a medium bowl and put into a large tightly sealed plastic bag. Marinate chicken at least 30 minutes or overnight in the refrigerator for best results.

6. Preheat grill to medium high and place chicken legs on grill grate. Cook as per directions for direct heat method (page 3), keeping in mind that the chicken legs will take between 20–25 minutes to cook through. (See Test Chicken for Doneness, page 21.)

SPICY SCALLOP "KISSES" WITH TARRAGON AND LEMON

SERVES: 6 SERVING SIZE: ¹/₆ recipe

I'm a seafood purist and when you combine pristine fresh scallops with simple ingredients, it allows the natural sweet flavor of the scallops to emerge. Delicate tarragon and fresh lemon bolster the scallops' flavor.

1¹/₂ pounds sea scallops

3 tablespoons fresh tarragon, minced

2 tablespoons chives, minced

1 tablespoon extra virgin olive oil

2 teaspoons salted butter, melted

Juice of 1 lemon

¹/₄ teaspoon cayenne pepper

2 slices cooked bacon, chopped (optional)

1. Combine all the ingredients in a mixing bowl.

2. Divide the scallops into 12-inch aluminum foil squares. Fold up the corners forming, loose pouches or pockets around the scallops.

3. Preheat grill to medium high and place scallop packets on grill grate. Cook as per directions for direct heat method (page 3), turning a few times during the 10–12-minute cooking time. This should be enough time to cook the shellfish through to doneness. They should be totally opaque once cooked through. Open the packets tableside in front of each person.

EXCHANGES
¹/₂ CARBOHYDRATE
2 LEAN MEAT

CALORIES 130
  CALORIES FROM FAT 40
TOTAL FAT 4.5 g
  SATURATED FAT 1.3 g
  TRANS FAT 0.1 g
CHOLESTEROL 40 mg
SODIUM 235 mg
POTASSIUM 295 mg
TOTAL CARBOHYDRATE 5 g
  DIETARY FIBER 0 g
  SUGARS 0 g
PROTEIN 18 g
PHOSPHORUS 365 mg

GRILLED TURKEY TACOS

SERVES: 6   **SERVING SIZE:** 1 taco   **MARINATING TIME:** At least 30 minutes or overnight

These tacos are quite delicious, and I personally prefer them instead of beef tacos. Using turkey brings out the flavor of the vegetables.

1 pound turkey tenderloin, sliced like a book through the center and lightly pounded out.

MARINADE

1 tablespoon canola oil
1 teaspoon oregano
1 teaspoon chili powder
1 teaspoon cumin
2 teaspoons unsweetened cocoa
1 jalapeño pepper, seeded and minced
  Juice of 1 lime

GARNISH

6 6-inch corn tortillas
¼ cup red onion, chopped
¼ cup tomatoes, chopped
1 cup cabbage, shredded
1 ripe avocado, chopped
½ cup fat-free Greek yogurt

1. Combine all of the marinade ingredients in a medium bowl and put into a large, tightly sealed plastic bag. Marinate turkey at least 30 minutes or overnight in the refrigerator for best results.

2. Preheat grill to medium high and place turkey on grill grate. Cook as per directions for direct heat method (page 3), keeping in mind that 10–12 minutes per side should be enough to cook the turkey through to doneness. (See Test Chicken for Doneness, page 21.) Set cooked turkey breast aside.

3. Slice or chop the grilled turkey and divide among the corn tortillas, which can be warmed in the microwave or in a dry sauté pan.

4. Garnish with onion, tomato, cabbage, avocado, and yogurt. You may also sprinkle with shredded cheddar or jack cheese before serving.

EXCHANGES
1 STARCH
3 LEAN MEAT

CALORIES 225
  CALORIES FROM FAT 65
TOTAL FAT 7.0 g
  SATURATED FAT 1.0 g
  TRANS FAT 0.0 g
CHOLESTEROL 50 mg
SODIUM 50 mg
POTASSIUM 460 mg
TOTAL CARBOHYDRATE 19 g
  DIETARY FIBER 4 g
  SUGARS 3 g
PROTEIN 22 g
PHOSPHORUS 270 mg

STEAKHOUSE SALAD WITH TOMATO AND CUCUMBER

SERVES: 4   **SERVING SIZE:** ¼ recipe   **MARINATING TIME:** At least 15 minutes or overnight

This entrée salad will please every member of the family, but it's great as a special meal with a warm loaf of bread. You can treat chicken breasts or shrimp with the same marinade and serve warm on the salad.

1 pound skirt steak or flank steak, well-trimmed.

MARINADE

1 tablespoon olive oil
1 teaspoon fresh thyme, minced
½ teaspoon fennel seeds
½ teaspoon black pepper, ground
1 tablespoon balsamic or sherry vinegar

SALAD

2 cucumbers, peeled if skin is thick, sliced ¼ inch thick
2 ripe medium tomatoes, sliced ¼ inch thick
½ cup red onion, thinly sliced
¾ cup low-fat gorgonzola or blue cheese, crumbled or sliced (optional)
2 tablespoons extra virgin olive oil
2 tablespoons red wine vinegar
½ teaspoon fresh ground black pepper
½ teaspoon kosher or sea salt

1. Combine all of the marinade ingredients in a medium bowl and put into a large tightly sealed plastic bag. Marinate at least 15 minutes at room temperature or overnight in the refrigerator for best results.

2. Preheat grill to medium high and place steak on grill grate. Cook as per directions for direct heat method (page 3), keeping in mind that 5–6 minutes per side should be enough to cook them completely through. Set aside. Cool 15 minutes before slicing against the grain about ¼ inch thick.

3. Mound the sliced vegetables on a platter. Sprinkle the cheese over the salad and drizzle with oil and vinegar. Season with pepper and salt.

EXCHANGES
2 VEGETABLE
3 LEAN MEAT
2 FAT

CALORIES 280
 CALORIES FROM FAT 145
TOTAL FAT 16.0 g
 SATURATED FAT 4.4 g
 TRANS FAT 0.0 g
CHOLESTEROL 75 mg
SODIUM 190 mg
POTASSIUM 615 mg
TOTAL CARBOHYDRATE 8 g
 DIETARY FIBER 2 g
 SUGARS 5 g
PROTEIN 26 g
PHOSPHORUS 260 mg

GRILLED EXOTIC MUSHROOM SALAD

SERVES: 5   **SERVING SIZE**: ¹/₅ recipe   **MARINATING TIME**: 20 minutes

If you love mushrooms, this is the recipe for you. I typically serve this salad over arugula or baby spinach.

6 ounces portabello mushrooms, whole
1 pound button mushrooms, whole
4 ounces shiitake mushrooms, whole, stem removed

MUSHROOM MARINADE
2 cloves garlic, minced
1 shallot, minced
1 tablespoon Dijon mustard
¼ cup olive oil
2 tablespoons balsamic vinegar
2 tablespoons tarragon, fresh, minced
1 tablespoon parsley, fresh, minced
   Freshly ground pepper from a mill
2 ounces sherry wine (optional)

1 16-ounce can cannellini beans (white kidney)
   drained, rinsed well
2 tablespoons toasted pine nuts (optional)

1. Combine all of the marinade ingredients in a medium bowl and put into a large tightly sealed plastic bag. Marinate for 20 minutes at room temperature. You can use the remaining marinade as a dressing for the salad.

2. Preheat grill to medium high and place mushrooms on grill grate. Cook as per directions for direct heat method (page 3), keeping in mind that 5–6 minutes should be enough to cook the mushrooms completely through. Set aside. Cool 15 minutes before slicing.

3. Slice the grilled mushrooms in ½-inch-thick slices and combine with the white beans. Moisten with some of the extra tarragon marinade and serve over mixed greens.

4. Garnish with toasted pine nuts.

EXCHANGES
1 STARCH
1 VEGETABLE
1 LEAN MEAT
1¹/₂ FAT

CALORIES 210
  CALORIES FROM FAT 110
TOTAL FAT 12.0 g
  SATURATED FAT 1.6 g
  TRANS FAT 0.0 g
CHOLESTEROL 0 mg
SODIUM 135 mg
POTASSIUM 750 mg
TOTAL CARBOHYDRATE 20 g
  DIETARY FIBER 5 g
  SUGARS 4 g
PROTEIN 9 g
PHOSPHORUS 220 mg

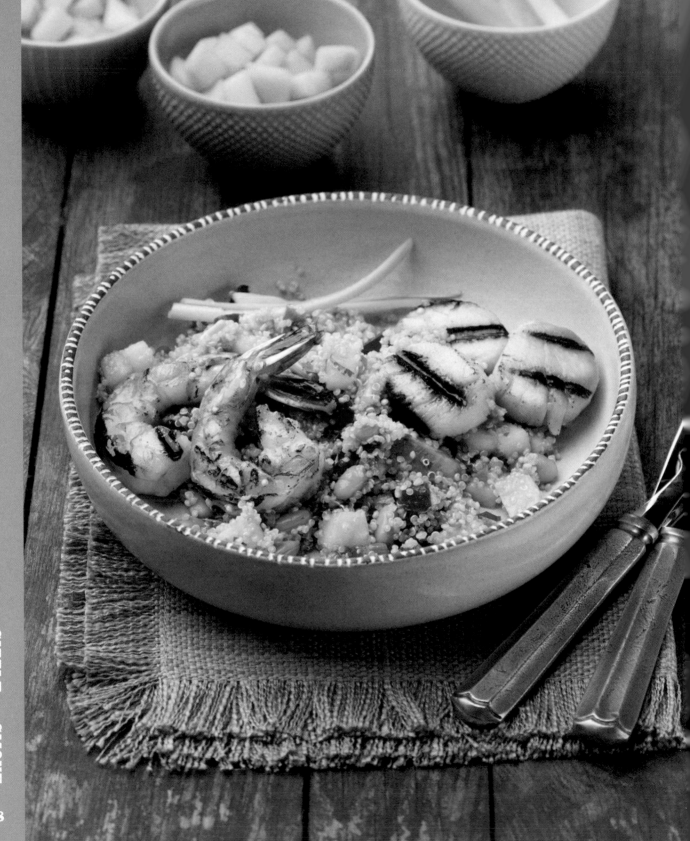

GRILLED SEAFOOD AND QUINOA SALAD WITH MANGO AND AVOCADO

SERVES: 4   **SERVING SIZE:** ¼ recipe   **MARINATING TIME:** At least 30 minutes or overnight

Latin American influence permeates this colorful recipe full of bold taste and textures. You can add any leftover cooked meats or seafood to this recipe as well.

CITRUS DRESSING

- 2 tablespoons fresh lime juice
- 2 tablespoons orange juice
- 1 teaspoon honey
- 1 tablespoon extra virgin olive oil
- Sea salt, to taste
- ¼ teaspoon cayenne pepper

- 1 cup dry quinoa, rinsed well
- ½ pound medium shrimp, peeled and deveined
- ½ pound scallops
- Olive oil (for marinating and brushing)
- ½ cup cooked black beans or edamame
- 1 jalapeño, stemmed and finely chopped
- ½ red bell pepper, chopped
- 1 plum tomato, seeded and chopped
- 2 small scallions, chopped
- 1 mango, chopped
- 1 avocado, chopped
- 2 tablespoons cilantro leaves, chopped
- Juice of 1 lime

1. Combine all citrus dressing ingredients well in a small mixing bowl.

2. Cook the quinoa according to directions in water. Fluff quinoa with a fork. If any liquid remains, continue simmering until it is absorbed. Let the quinoa cool completely.

3. Toss the shrimp and scallops with the olive oil in a bowl.

4. Heat a grill pan or sauté pan over medium-high heat. Add the shrimp and scallops and sear until pink and just cooked through, about 2 minutes per side. Remove from the pan and let cool.

5. Place the cooled quinoa in a large bowl and add the shrimp and scallops, beans, jalapeño, bell pepper, tomato, scallions, mango, and avocado. Pour the dressing over the mixture and toss gently to combine.

6. Divide the salad among four plates or bowls and scatter cilantro leaves over each.

EXCHANGES	
2½ STARCH	
1 FRUIT	
1 VEGETABLE	
3 LEAN MEAT	
1½ FAT	

CALORIES 470	
CALORIES FROM FAT 145	
TOTAL FAT 16.0 g	
SATURATED FAT 2.4 g	
TRANS FAT 0.0 g	
CHOLESTEROL 110 mg	
SODIUM 315 mg	
POTASSIUM 1020 mg	
TOTAL CARBOHYDRATE 56 g	
DIETARY FIBER 10 g	
SUGARS 16 g	
PROTEIN 30 g	
PHOSPHORUS 565 mg	

TERRA COTTA CHICKEN COBB SALAD WITH SPICY LIME DRIZZLE

SERVES: 3 **SERVING SIZE**: ¹/₃ recipe

This is a really wonderful way to use leftover grilled chicken breasts. For an attractive presentation, arrange rows of colorful ingredients over top of salad before drizzling with dressing.

SALAD

- 8 ounces cooked chicken breast, chopped
- ¹/₂ red pepper, chopped
- ¹/₂ green pepper, chopped
- ¹/₄ red onion, chopped
- 1 medium tomato, chopped
- ¹/₂ avocado, chopped
- ¹/₄ cup reduced-fat blue cheese, low fat
- 1 hardboiled egg, chopped
- 2 cups packed salad greens, such as baby field greens, romaine, arugula, spinach, or any favorite blend

LIME DRIZZLE

- 2 teaspoons extra virgin olive oil
- ¹/₄ cup low-fat buttermilk
- 2 teaspoons jarred pickled jalapeño, minced
  Juice of 1 lime
- 2 teaspoons Dijon mustard

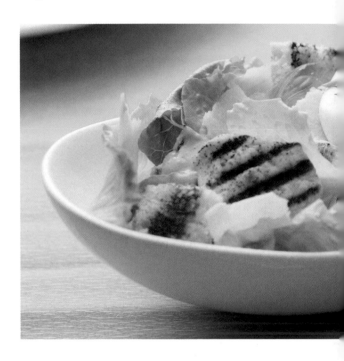

1. Combine all salad ingredients in a large mixing bowl.

2. Combine lime drizzle ingredients and pour over salad right before serving.

EXCHANGES
2 VEGETABLE
4 LEAN MEAT
1 FAT

CALORIES 290
  CALORIES FROM FAT 115
TOTAL FAT 13.0 g
  SATURATED FAT 3.5 g
  TRANS FAT 0.0 g
CHOLESTEROL 130 mg
SODIUM 330 mg
POTASSIUM 705 mg
TOTAL CARBOHYDRATE 12 g
  DIETARY FIBER 4 g
  SUGARS 5 g
PROTEIN 31 g
PHOSPHORUS 310 mg

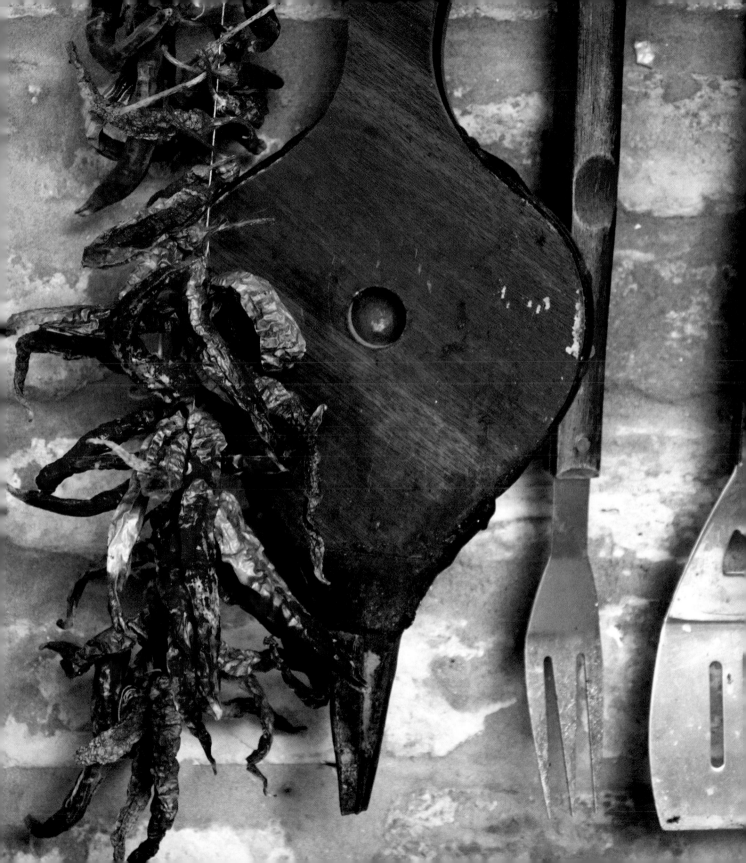

CHAPTER 3
Over the Top

No matter what kind of grill master you may be, what separates the masters from the beginners are grill toppers. What I mean by this is that great grilled food is a natural canvas for all kinds of delicious salsas, chutneys, sauces, or drizzles. There are some distinct advantages to grill toppers. They can often be made a few days in advance and become even better as the flavors mingle.

Many of the recipes in this chapter add color and interest as well and can be used for many other recipes. Most of these recipes double as a spread for sandwiches and Bruschetta. Some recipes, such as the Greek Yogurt Raita (page 87), are meant to cool down the flavor of impending spice, while other recipes, like the Romesco Sauce (page 88) or Chimmi-Churri Sauce (page 89) were designed for a rush of taste against a mild piece of grilled chicken, tofu, or seafood. I have to tell you that the Romesco Sauce, Chimmi-Churri Sauce, and Satay Peanut Sauce (page 89) recipes are my favorite all-time sauces to serve whenever I fire up the grill. I usually make double batches and then eat them all week on everything from salads to crudités, along with grilled or steamed dishes.

On the salsa side, I'm kind of over regular tomato salsa. As a result, I offer you some wonderful alternatives, such as Feta Tomato Salsa (page 95) (originally made for a supermarket chain I worked for), or Double Apple Pomegranate (page 84), a fall/winter favorite. Shakshuka (page 90) was introduced to me by my fiancée, Lori, who lived in Israel and was married to a Moroccan man. Apparently, this continues to be a controversial rendition because it's such a classic in each country throughout the Middle East. My version was created with a more modern American twist.

It seems like everyone is getting back to making their own pickles in restaurants everywhere I go. Originally, these vegetables were developed for the Bahn Mi Sandwich (page 70). I now keep a jar in my fridge and find them especially fulfilling when I'm trying to drop a few pounds, as I can eat loads of them somewhat guiltlessly. In a few weeks, you are sure to identify your favorites, which I hope you incorporate into your go-to list of favorite grill toppers.

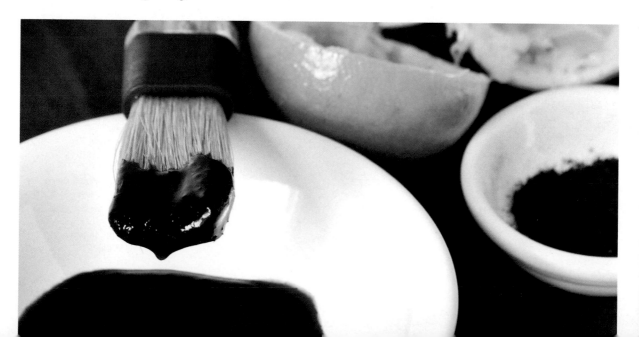

DOUBLE APPLE-POMEGRANATE SALSA

SERVES: 6   SERVING SIZE: 2 ounces

Crispy, juicy, tart, spicy, and lightly sweet from agave, this is a salsa that energizes anything from the grill or broiler. It's also wonderful on sandwiches and grilled sausages.

- 2 apples, unpeeled, such as Granny Smith, Gala, Fuji, or Pink Lady, diced into 1/2-inch cubes
  Juice of 1 lemon
- 1 tablespoon honey or agave syrup
- 1 tablespoon brown sugar
- 1 jalapeño pepper, seeded, minced
- 1 cup fresh pomegranate seeds
- 1/4 cup dried apples, chopped
- 1/4 cup pomegranate juice, such as Pom

1. Combine all ingredients in a medium mixing bowl and allow to marinate for at least a half hour or overnight in the refrigerator.

EXCHANGES
1 1/2 FRUIT

CALORIES 90
 CALORIES FROM FAT 5
TOTAL FAT 0.5 g
 SATURATED FAT 0.1 g
 TRANS FAT 0.0 g
CHOLESTEROL 0 mg
SODIUM 10 mg
POTASSIUM 200 mg
TOTAL CARBOHYDRATE 23 g
 DIETARY FIBER 3 g
 SUGARS 18 g
PROTEIN 1 g
PHOSPHORUS 25 mg

MINESTRONE GARDEN RELISH

SERVES: 4   SERVING SIZE: 1/4 recipe

This recipe is fresh, light, and super colorful, whether it's over any grilled protein, cooked pasta, rice, or even a baked potato. It's really spectacular on sandwiches as well.

- 1 cup chopped ripe tomato
- 1 cup diced zucchini
- 1/2 cup canned chopped artichoke hearts, drained
- 1/2 cup chopped fresh basil
- 1/3 cup diced bottled roasted red bell peppers
- 1/4 cup minced red onion
- 2 tablespoons chopped pitted Kalamata olives
- 1 tablespoon balsamic vinegar
- 2 teaspoons olive oil
- 1/2 teaspoon crushed red chili flakes

1. Combine all ingredients in a medium mixing bowl and allow to marinate for 20 minutes before serving.

EXCHANGES
2 VEGETABLE
1 FAT

CALORIES 80
 CALORIES FROM FAT 35
TOTAL FAT 4.0 g
 SATURATED FAT 0.5 g
 TRANS FAT 0.0 g
CHOLESTEROL 0 mg
SODIUM 180 mg
POTASSIUM 330 mg
TOTAL CARBOHYDRATE 9 g
 DIETARY FIBER 3 g
 SUGARS 4 g
PROTEIN 2 g
PHOSPHORUS 50 mg

FLORIDA SOFRITO

SERVES: 32   **SERVING SIZE:** 2 tablespoons

There are so many variations of Sofrito, which is a Latin or Caribbean-based seasoning condiment. You can add it to rice, pasta, beans, or even as a seasoning to marinate meat, poultry, or seafood before grilling. This version is cooked, while others are left raw. You can leave this Sofrito chopped or purée it with a hand-held immersion blender or in a food processor. Keep it in a covered jar refrigerated for up to a week. You may also freeze it in ice cube trays and pull out what you need as you need it.

1 tablespoon olive oil

1 medium Spanish onion, chopped

2 large tomatoes, halved, seeds squeezed out, and chopped

1 small green bell pepper, seeded and chopped

1 red pepper, seeded and chopped

1 jalapeño or serrano chili, seeded and chopped

3 cloves garlic, minced

2 teaspoons ground cumin

2 teaspoons dried oregano

1 tablespoon tomato paste

1 cup cilantro leaves, chopped

1. Heat oil over medium heat in a large saucepot. Sauté the onion, tomato, peppers, chili, garlic, cumin, and oregano for 5 minutes, stirring frequently.

2. Add the tomato paste and continue to cook until the tomato paste caramelizes and turns light brown. Add the cilantro and combine well. Cool and refrigerate for later use.

EXCHANGES
FREE FOOD

CALORIES 10
  CALORIES FROM FAT 5
TOTAL FAT 0.5 g
  SATURATED FAT 0.1 g
  TRANS FAT 0.0 g
CHOLESTEROL 0 mg
SODIUM 5 mg
POTASSIUM 65 mg
TOTAL CARBOHYDRATE 2 g
  DIETARY FIBER 0 g
  SUGARS 1 g
PROTEIN 0 g
PHOSPHORUS 10 mg

HAITIAN CHILI LIME SAUCE

SERVES: 32   **SERVING SIZE**: 2 tablespoons

This is a wonderful marinade or seasoning condiment that can top off any grilled beef, poultry, or seafood dish. Just a few spoonfuls go a really long way in the flavor department. You can keep it for weeks covered in your refrigerator. During chili pepper season, I often make jars of this as gifts for friends.

1 large red onion, thinly sliced
6 scallions, thinly sliced
3 cloves garlic, thinly sliced
½ cup lime juice
¼ cup white vinegar
¼ cup water
3 sprigs fresh thyme, leave on the branch
1 hot pepper, either jalapeño, Scotch bonnet, or serrano, thinly sliced
2 tablespoons olive oil

1. Bring all ingredients to a boil. Immediately remove from the stove and cool.

EXCHANGES
FREE FOOD

CALORIES 15
  CALORIES FROM FAT 10
TOTAL FAT 1.0 g
  SATURATED FAT 0.1 g
  TRANS FAT 0.0 g
CHOLESTEROL 0 mg
SODIUM 0 mg
POTASSIUM 25 mg
TOTAL CARBOHYDRATE 1 g
  DIETARY FIBER 0 g
  SUGARS 0 g
PROTEIN 0 g
PHOSPHORUS 0 mg

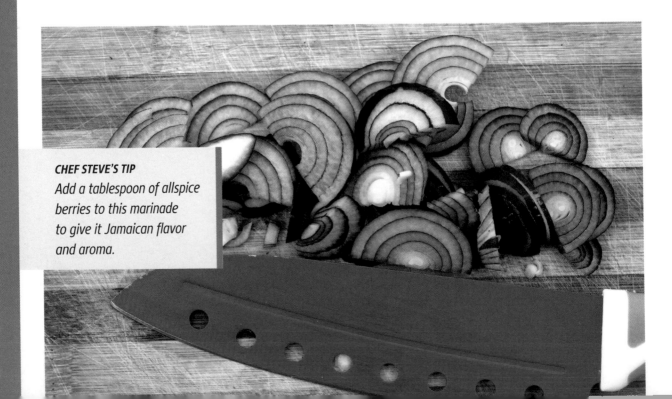

CHEF STEVE'S TIP
Add a tablespoon of allspice berries to this marinade to give it Jamaican flavor and aroma.

SOUTH MAPLE RUM PEPPER DRIZZLE

SERVES: 16   **SERVING SIZE:** 2 tablespoons

This is a somewhat sophisticated sauce to lightly drizzle over grilled steaks, chops, and poultry. It's also great over sweet potatoes and butternut squash.

1 tablespoon butter, unsalted
1 tablespoon olive oil
2 large shallots, minced
$^1/_2$ cup dark rum
2 cups beef, chicken, or vegetable stock
$^1/_2$ teaspoon black pepper, coarsely milled
1 tablespoon maple syrup

1. Heat butter and oil in a medium saucepot over medium heat. Add shallots and sauté for 1 minute until they soften.

2. Add rum and reduce the liquid by half. Add the stock, pepper, and maple syrup and simmer for 10 minutes until lightly thickened.

EXCHANGES
$^1/_2$ FAT

CALORIES 30
  CALORIES FROM FAT 15
TOTAL FAT 1.5 g
  SATURATED FAT 0.6 g
  TRANS FAT 0.0 g
CHOLESTEROL 0 mg
SODIUM 110 mg
POTASSIUM 30 mg
TOTAL CARBOHYDRATE 2 g
  DIETARY FIBER 0 g
  SUGARS 1 g
PROTEIN 0 g
PHOSPHORUS 5 mg

GREEK YOGURT RAITA

SERVES: 12   **SERVING SIZE:** $^1/_4$ cup

Bold in flavor and a beautiful golden color, this turns the simplest grilled item into exotic fare. I like it on grilled eggplant slabs and over grilled tofu and lamb chops as it stands up to all.

1 (16-ounce) carton plain, fat-free Greek yogurt
1 cup chopped seeded, peeled cucumber
1 cup chopped seeded tomato
$^1/_2$ cup minced red onion
$^1/_4$ cup fresh minced mint
$^1/_4$ cup fresh minced cilantro
1 teaspoon ground curry powder
$^1/_2$ teaspoon salt

1. Combine all ingredients in a medium mixing bowl and allow to marinate for 20 minutes before serving.

EXCHANGES
1 VEGETABLE

CALORIES 30
  CALORIES FROM FAT 0
TOTAL FAT 0.0 g
  SATURATED FAT 0.0 g
  TRANS FAT 0.0 g
CHOLESTEROL 0 mg
SODIUM 115 mg
POTASSIUM 115 mg
TOTAL CARBOHYDRATE 3 g
  DIETARY FIBER 1 g
  SUGARS 2 g
PROTEIN 4 g
PHOSPHORUS 60 mg

ROMESCO SAUCE

SERVES: 8 **SERVING SIZE**: ¹/₈ recipe

This incredible sauce goes with everything and is probably my favorite sauce to serve for guests. I serve it with grilled or raw vegetables, grilled meats, or as a sandwich spread and people always ask for the recipe. Now they have it!

- 1 8-ounce jar roasted red peppers, drained well
- 1 medium tomato, ripe, chopped, or 1 cup tomatoes in juice, drained well
- 3 garlic cloves, peeled
- ¹/₂ teaspoon crushed red chili flakes
- 1 tablespoon smoked paprika
- 2 tablespoons tomato paste
- ¹/₄ cup panko breadcrumbs or dried, stale bread, torn and soaked in water
- ¹/₂ cup almonds, sliced or whole
- 2 tablespoons sherry or balsamic vinegar
- ¹/₂ teaspoon kosher salt

1. Process all ingredients in a food processor or blender until smooth.

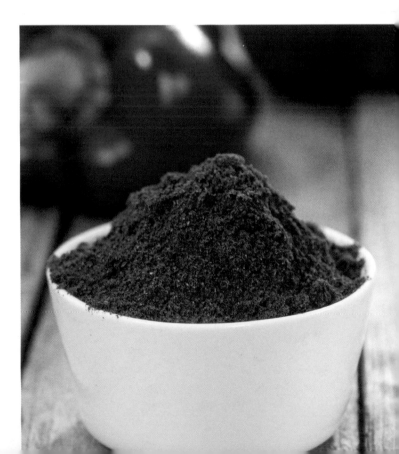

EXCHANGES
¹/₂ CARBOHYDRATE
¹/₂ FAT

CALORIES 55
  CALORIES FROM FAT 25
TOTAL FAT 3.0 g
  SATURATED FAT 0.3 g
  TRANS FAT 0.0 g
CHOLESTEROL 0 mg
SODIUM 180 mg
POTASSIUM 185 mg
TOTAL CARBOHYDRATE 6 g
  DIETARY FIBER 2 g
  SUGARS 2 g
PROTEIN 2 g
PHOSPHORUS 45 mg

SATAY PEANUT SAUCE

SERVES: 14   **SERVING SIZE**: $1/14$ recipe

This is one of my absolute favorite recipes. I enjoy it on almost everything.

10 ounces water
 1 tablespoon ginger root, mined
$1/2$ teaspoon crushed red chili flakes
$3/4$ cup chunky peanut butter
 1 tablespoon brown sugar
 1 tablespoon reduced-sodium soy sauce
 1 tablespoon tomato catsup
 1 tablespoon lime juice
$1/4$ cup cilantro, minced

1. Place all ingredients except cilantro in a medium saucepan and bring to a simmer. Combine well with a whisk until smooth and simmer for 5 minutes. Adjust tartness if necessary and make it spicier if you prefer. Add cilantro.

EXCHANGES
2 FAT

CALORIES 90
 CALORIES FROM FAT 65
TOTAL FAT 7.0 g
 SATURATED FAT 1.4 g
 TRANS FAT 0.0 g
CHOLESTEROL 0 mg
SODIUM 120 mg
POTASSIUM 90 mg
TOTAL CARBOHYDRATE 4 g
 DIETARY FIBER 1 g
 SUGARS 2 g
PROTEIN 4 g
PHOSPHORUS 50 mg

CHIMMI-CHURRI SAUCE

SERVES: 16   **SERVING SIZE**: 1 tablespoon

This sauce can be made with parsley, basil, or any favorite herb if you are not a cilantro fan. It's wonderful on grilled tofu, tempeh, or any grilled vegetable steak. Try it on a grilled vegetable sandwich on a fresh ciabatta roll or French bread.

 2 cups packed cilantro leaves
$1/2$ cup packed flat-leaf parsley
 3 cloves garlic
 3 scallions
$1/2$ cup extra-virgin olive oil
 1 jalapeño pepper, seeded and chopped
 2 teaspoons kosher salt
    Juice of 1 lime

1. Wash cilantro and parsley. Place all ingredients in a blender or food processor fitted with metal blade and process 45 seconds or until combined well.

EXCHANGES
$1 1/2$ FAT

CALORIES 65
 CALORIES FROM FAT 65
TOTAL FAT 7.0 g
 SATURATED FAT 0.9 g
 TRANS FAT 0.0 g
CHOLESTEROL 0 mg
SODIUM 235 mg
POTASSIUM 35 mg
TOTAL CARBOHYDRATE 1 g
 DIETARY FIBER 0 g
 SUGARS 0 g
PROTEIN 0 g
PHOSPHORUS 0 mg

SHAKSHUKA

SERVES: 5   **SERVING SIZE**: ¹/₅ recipe

My fiancée lived in Israel for many years and this seems to be the go-to dish for many of her friends. It can be eaten at any meal, late at night, or as a snack. You can leave the eggs out if you prefer and just enjoy it as a soul-warming sauce for grilled seafood, poultry, or meat.

1 tablespoon extra virgin olive oil

1 medium Spanish onion, diced

2 cloves garlic, minced

1 medium green or red bell pepper, chopped

1 jalapeño pepper, seeded and minced

1 teaspoon cumin, ground

1 teaspoon chili powder

1 teaspoon smoked paprika

2 tablespoons tomato paste

4 cups ripe diced tomatoes, or 2 cans (14 ounces each) diced tomatoes in juice

5 eggs

¹/₂ tablespoon fresh chopped parsley

1. Heat oil in a large, heavy-bottomed sauté pan with raised sides, preferably a black iron Griswold or Le Creuset ware, over medium heat.

2. Sauté onion, garlic, bell pepper, and jalapeño for 3-4 minutes until softened. Add all the spices and sauté for a minute to expand the flavor of the spice.

3. Add the tomato paste and continue to sauté until the paste begins to color, stirring constantly. Add the tomatoes and combine well, stirring to distribute the paste well. Simmer for 7–9 minutes until a sauce forms and it thickens.

4. Crack the eggs over the tomato mixture gently and space them evenly around the pan. Cover the pan and gently simmer for 5–7 minutes until the eggs are cooked through, but leave the yolk a bit runny.

EXCHANGES
2 VEGETABLE
1 MED-FAT MEAT
¹/₂ FAT

CALORIES 135
  CALORIES FROM FAT 70
TOTAL FAT 8.0 g
  SATURATED FAT 2.0 g
  TRANS FAT 0.0 g
CHOLESTEROL 185 mg
SODIUM 140 mg
POTASSIUM 635 mg
TOTAL CARBOHYDRATE 13 g
  DIETARY FIBER 4 g
  SUGARS 7 g
PROTEIN 9 g
PHOSPHORUS 165 mg

POLONAISE PARSLEY AND EGG CRUMBLE

SERVES: 6 **SERVING SIZE**: ¹/₆ recipe

I learned this recipe while attending the Culinary Institute of America many years ago. It's a classic French garnish normally served over steamed or grilled vegetables such as asparagus, broccoli, or green beans. And I understand why it's timeless. It's perfect for the family dinner table or company.

2 tablespoons no-trans fat, nonhydrogenated buttery spread (such as Smart Balance), melted

¹/₂ cup breadcrumbs, unseasoned

2 hardboiled eggs, chopped

¹/₄ cup parsley, minced

1 teaspoon lemon zest

¹/₂ teaspoon kosher or sea salt

1 tablespoon Parmesan cheese, shredded (optional)

1. Heat butter in a saucepan over medium-high heat. Add breadcrumbs and toast lightly. Add the eggs, parsley, lemon zest, salt, and Parmesan cheese, if using.

2. Fold into your favorite vegetable while still warm.

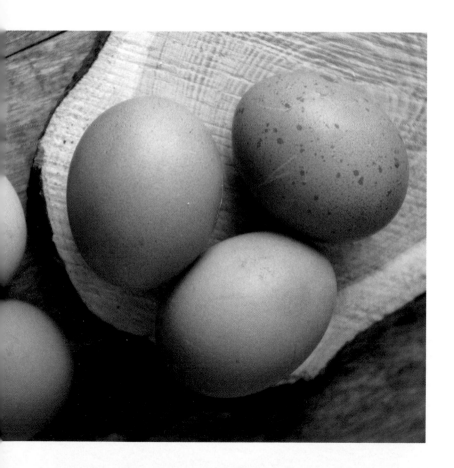

EXCHANGES
¹/₂ STARCH
1 FAT

CALORIES 85
  CALORIES FROM FAT 45
TOTAL FAT 5.0 g
  SATURATED FAT 1.5 g
  TRANS FAT 0.0 g
CHOLESTEROL 60 mg
SODIUM 275 mg
POTASSIUM 55 mg
TOTAL CARBOHYDRATE 7 g
  DIETARY FIBER 1 g
  SUGARS 1 g
PROTEIN 3 g
PHOSPHORUS 50 mg

BASIL WALNUT RICOTTA PESTO

SERVES: 16   **SERVING SIZE**: 2 tablespoons

Not your typical pesto. You can add any fresh herbs to the pesto, such as oregano, mint, or tarragon. The ricotta cheese allows you to cut back on the oil a bit as well. I love this over grilled poultry, vegetable steaks, or mixed into whole-wheat spaghetti or penne.

4 cups whole basil leaves

¼ cup chopped chives or scallions

2 cloves garlic, peeled

1 jalapeño pepper, seeded

2 tablespoons pine nuts

2 tablespoons walnuts

3 tablespoons low-fat ricotta cheese

2 tablespoons good-quality Parmesan or Romano cheese

¼ cup extra-virgin olive oil

Salt, to taste

1. Purée all ingredients in a food processor fitted with the metal blade or in a blender for a few moments until smooth, creamy, and bright green.

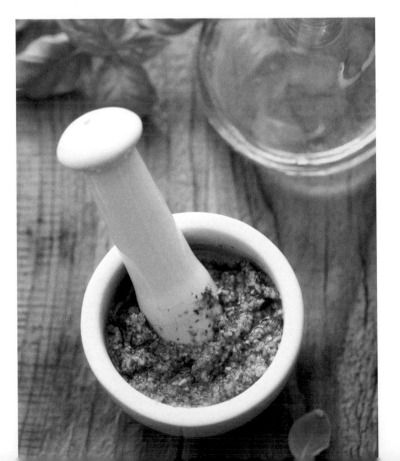

EXCHANGES
2 FAT

CALORIES 55
  CALORIES FROM FAT 45
TOTAL FAT 5.0 g
  SATURATED FAT 0.7 g
  TRANS FAT 0.0 g
CHOLESTEROL 0 mg
SODIUM 15 mg
POTASSIUM 80 mg
TOTAL CARBOHYDRATE 1 g
  DIETARY FIBER 1 g
  SUGARS 0 g
PROTEIN 1 g
PHOSPHORUS 30 mg

OLIVE AND FIG TAPENADE

SERVES: 32   **SERVING SIZE**: 1 tablespoon

This take on classic tapenade was developed by my chef friend Brian Morris. We prepared this tapenade in front of thousands of home cooks around the country as part of a national cooking show we performed together. The crowds always loved this recipe, which is wonderful spread on toasted bread rounds, over grilled poultry, or dipped into with crispy apples.

½ cup halved dried figs
1 cup water
2 garlic cloves, peeled
1 cup whole pitted black olives, drained
½ cup artichoke hearts, drained
1 tablespoon capers, rinsed and drained
1 tablespoon sherry or red wine vinegar
1 tablespoon orange zest
1 teaspoon fresh thyme leaves
¼ teaspoon black pepper
½ cup extra virgin olive oil

1. Place figs in a microwave-safe measuring cup and cover with cold water. Microwave on high 4 minutes, or until water is near boiling. Let cool at room temperature, allowing figs to soften. Drain and reserve 2 tablespoons of the soaking liquid.

2. Combine figs and reserved liquid with remaining ingredients, except olive oil, in a food processor. Process until smooth, or leave it chunkier to suit your taste.

3. With the motor running, drizzle in olive oil. Transfer to an airtight container and store in the refrigerator.

EXCHANGES
1 FAT

CALORIES 45
  CALORIES FROM FAT 35
TOTAL FAT 4.0 g
  SATURATED FAT 0.5 g
  TRANS FAT 0.0 g
CHOLESTEROL 0 mg
SODIUM 55 mg
POTASSIUM 25 mg
TOTAL CARBOHYDRATE 2 g
  DIETARY FIBER 1 g
  SUGARS 1 g
PROTEIN 0 g
PHOSPHORUS 0 mg

ANDALUCÍA-STYLE SEVILLE SAUCE

SERVES: 10   **SERVING SIZE**: ¹/₁₀ recipe

This sauce pops with sunshine and warmth. I serve it with grilled seafood and poultry. It's also incredible over grilled eggplant steaks, tofu, and tempeh spears.

1 cup whole garlic cloves, peeled
¹/₂ cup olive or canola oil
¹/₂ teaspoon kosher or sea salt
1 cup orange juice
2 tablespoons lime juice
2 teaspoons smoked paprika
¹/₂ teaspoon crushed red pepper flakes
¹/₄ cup fresh chopped parsley
1 teaspoon unsalted butter (optional)

1. Scatter garlic cloves in roast pan, cover with oil and sprinkle with salt. Roast in 375°F oven, stirring occasionally, for 18–20 minutes until golden and soft. Set aside.

2. Pour orange juice into a medium saucepot and reduce by half. Add all remaining ingredients, including roasted garlic cloves, and simmer for 3 minutes more.

EXCHANGES
¹/₂ CARBOHYDRATE
2 FAT

CALORIES 130
  CALORIES FROM FAT 100
TOTAL FAT 11.0 g
  SATURATED FAT 1.5 g
  TRANS FAT 0.0 g
CHOLESTEROL 0 mg
SODIUM 95 mg
POTASSIUM 125 mg
TOTAL CARBOHYDRATE
  8 g
  DIETARY FIBER 1 g
  SUGARS 2 g
PROTEIN 1 g
PHOSPHORUS 30 mg

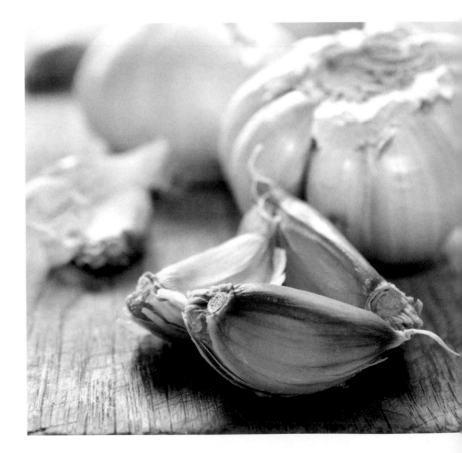

WISH I WAS ON THE BEACH TROPICAL FRUIT SALSA

SERVES: 8   SERVING SIZE: ⅛ recipe

Great over any grilled dish. Close your eyes, eat your first bite of grilled snapper with this salsa over the top, and presto, you'll feel like you're lounging on your favorite beach!

- ½ cup pineapple, diced
- ½ cup mango or papaya, diced
- ½ cup tomato, diced
- ½ cup water chestnuts, drained well and diced
- ¼ cup red pepper, diced
- 1 teaspoon ginger root, minced
- 2 teaspoons jalapeño, seeded and minced
- ¼ cup scallions, sliced
- 2 teaspoons lime juice

1. Combine all salad ingredients and mix well. If possible, allow to rest for at least 20 minutes before serving for the flavors to marry.

EXCHANGES
½ CARBOHYDRATE

CALORIES 20
  CALORIES FROM FAT 0
TOTAL FAT 0.0 g
  SATURATED FAT 0.0 g
  TRANS FAT 0.0 g
CHOLESTEROL 0 mg
SODIUM 0 mg
POTASSIUM 95 mg
TOTAL CARBOHYDRATE 5 g
  DIETARY FIBER 1 g
  SUGARS 3 g
PROTEIN 0 g
PHOSPHORUS 10 mg

FETA TOMATO SALSA

SERVES: 10   SERVING SIZE: ¼ cup

This salsa represents the true taste of the Mediterranean. You can serve it over any grilled item, plus it's also an amazing spread on a sandwich. Go ahead and try it over sliced cucumbers as a side salad.

- ½ cup reduced-fat feta crumbles
- 1 cup tomato, diced
- ¼ cup red onion, minced
- ¼ cup pitted kalamata olives, minced
- 1 tablespoon fresh oregano, minced
- ¼ cup fresh parsley, minced
- 1 tablespoon fresh dill, minced
- 2 tablespoons extra virgin olive oil

1. Combine all ingredients well in a small mixing bowl and allow to rest for at least 20 minutes for the flavors to marry.

EXCHANGES
1 FAT

CALORIES 55
  CALORIES FROM FAT 45
TOTAL FAT 5.0 g
  SATURATED FAT 1.0 g
  TRANS FAT 0.0 g
CHOLESTEROL 5 mg
SODIUM 140 mg
POTASSIUM 65 mg
TOTAL CARBOHYDRATE 2 g
  DIETARY FIBER 1 g
  SUGARS 1 g
PROTEIN 2 g
PHOSPHORUS 30 mg

HEARTS OF PALM AND AVOCADO SALAD

SERVES: 4   **SERVING SIZE**: ¼ recipe

Hearts of palm come both jarred and canned. I always prefer jarred in water so I can flavor them myself. This is a recipe from Costa Rica, where hearts of palm are plentiful. I love it over grilled entrees or served in a large goblet as an appetizer.

6–8 each jarred hearts of palm, rinsed and thinly sliced
¼ cup red onion, minced
½ cup red pepper, minced
1 tablespoon extra virgin olive oil
Juice of 1 lime
½ teaspoon kosher salt
⅛ teaspoon cayenne pepper
1 medium potato, peeled, cooked, and diced
1 large avocado, diced
2 tablespoons cilantro, minced

1. Combine all ingredients, adding the avocado and cilantro last. Serve in a wine glass or goblet.

EXCHANGES
1 CARBOHYDRATE
2 FAT

CALORIES 165
  CALORIES FROM FAT 90
TOTAL FAT 10.0 g
  SATURATED FAT 1.4 g
  TRANS FAT 0.0 g
CHOLESTEROL 0 mg
SODIUM 375 mg
POTASSIUM 1320 mg
TOTAL CARBOHYDRATE
  17 g
  DIETARY FIBER 5 g
  SUGARS 5 g
PROTEIN 4 g
PHOSPHORUS 115 mg

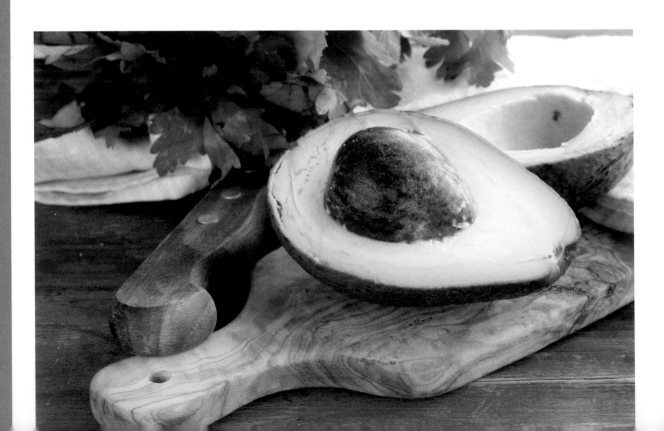

PICKLED VEGETABLES

SERVES: 16   **SERVING SIZE**: $^1/_{16}$ recipe

Pickles and pickled vegetables are a huge trend nationally. I've been making this island version for years. Throughout the Caribbean you can find a jar of these spicy pickled vegetables on every dining table. If you like a milder version, use half the amount of chili peppers or use a milder chili like a jalapeño or serrano.

4 Scotch bonnet peppers, stems trimmed and each pepper cut into 4 pieces

2 cups thin-sliced or shredded cabbage

$^1/_2$ cup thin-sliced or shredded carrots

$^1/_4$ cup thin-sliced or shredded onions

$^1/_4$ cup frozen green peas

4 whole cloves

2 bay leaves

6 allspice berries

1 teaspoon salt

3 cups white or cider vinegar

1. Place hot peppers, cabbage, carrots, onions, green peas, cloves, bay leaves, allspice berries, and salt in a clean 1-quart jar.

2. Add vinegar. Close jar tightly and let sit 24 to 48 hours. Then they are ready for use. Store refrigerated for up to 1 month.

EXCHANGES
FREE FOOD

CALORIES 15
  CALORIES FROM FAT 0
TOTAL FAT 0.0 g
  SATURATED FAT 0.0 g
  TRANS FAT 0.0 g
CHOLESTEROL 0 mg
SODIUM 80 mg
POTASSIUM 70 mg
TOTAL CARBOHYDRATE 3 g
  DIETARY FIBER 1 g
  SUGARS 1 g
PROTEIN 1 g
PHOSPHORUS 15 mg

CHAPTER 4
Sidekicks

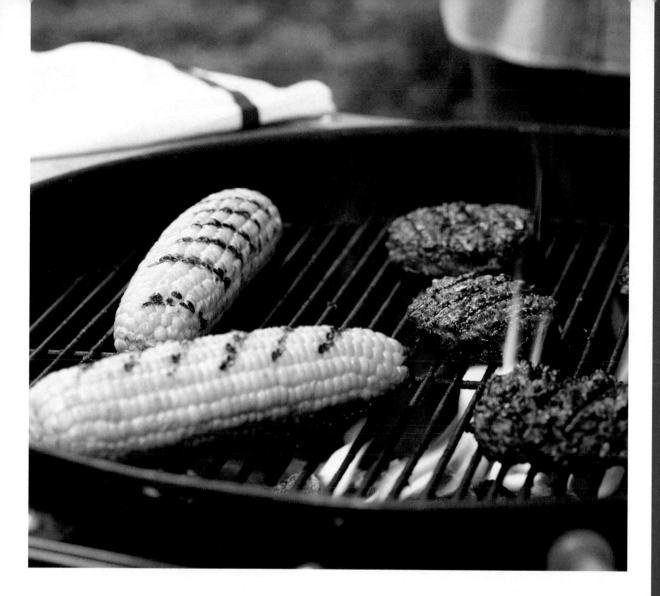

Like any other perfect relationship, the entrée and accompanying side dishes are more powerful together than any one is alone. They complement and perfect one another on the plate. That's what this chapter is all about. Whether grouped as a vegetarian dinner or used to accompany a favorite entrée, these are all unique recipes that can either stand alone or form a great team.

This chapter reflects authentic global dishes and quiet regional American sides that stick out from the pack. With the availability of international ingredients, crafted spice mixtures, infused oils and vinegars, and exotic salts, simple meals are easily transformed into something very special. Fresh seasonal asparagus pairs so well with truffle salt and Parmesan. Side dishes are very personal and they represent a menu category that allows for playfulness and experimentation. It's also totally acceptable to combine different ethnic dishes, as well as marinated salads, cooked vegetables, grains, pasta, legumes, and even plantains without criticism or scrutiny.

AN ASPARAGUS PRIMER— THE PERFECT PARTNER FOR ANY GRILLED DISH

If Oscar nominations or Emmy awards were given out for the most accomplished vegetable, asparagus would certainly win hands down. Delicate in flavor, it pairs nicely with many toppings and flavor add-ons. Here are some of the best ways to prepare the queen of the produce world. Any of the following cooking methods work with the toppings listed.

- COOKING METHODS | Steamed, roasted, on the grill, in a grill pan, or stir-fried. If roasting in an oven or grilling in a pan, it works best to blanch the asparagus first for 2 minutes in boiling water. Right after boiling, plunge it into ice-cold water, which is called 'shocking.' This process opens up the pores of the vegetable, allowing any marinate or spice to penetrate and cook into the stems.

- "FLAVOR DRIZZLES" | Select an oil, such as extra virgin olive oil, sesame oil, walnut oil, truffle oil, hazelnut oil, or corn oil. Combine oil with any vinegar, such as white wine, balsamic, raspberry, rice, apple cider, pomegranate, fig, or herb vinegar in the ratio of 3 parts oil to 1 part vinegar. Add salt and pepper and drizzle over asparagus.

- POLONAISE | 2 chopped hardboiled eggs, $1/4$ cup breadcrumbs, $1/4$ cup chopped parsley, $1/4$ cup olive oil, and 2 cloves minced garlic.

- NUTS | Chopped nuts of any kind are fabulous, especially if you brown them in a bit of olive oil for 2 minutes until golden brown. Use 8–10 chopped almonds, walnuts, pecans, pine nuts, hazelnuts, or cashews—they all work well. Serves 4.

- SEEDS | Place sesame, poppy, mustard, caraway, or black sesame seeds in a dry pan and toss over the heat for a minute to expand the flavor. Sprinkle over the asparagus spears.

- CHEESE | A delicate sprinkle of Parmesan, Manchego, Romano, queso blanco, or feta is incredible along with a drizzle of extra virgin olive oil and cracked pepper.

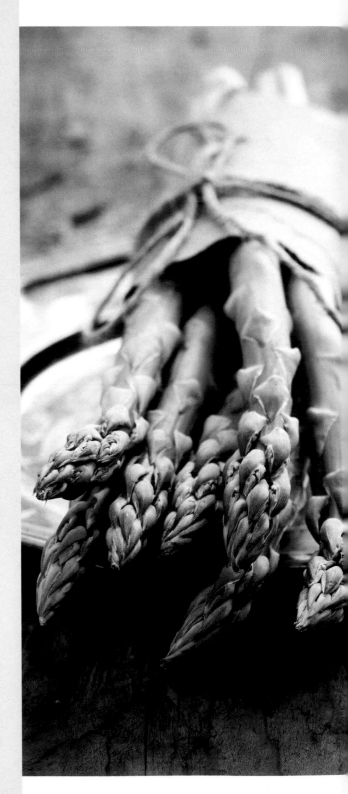

RAINBOW CONFETTI QUINOA

SERVES: 8   SERVING SIZE: ⅛ recipe

Super food and high-protein grain, quinoa is elegant and can be made days ahead of serving. You can even have a pile of this with spicy black beans on top and consider it a great dinner on its own.

2 teaspoons extra virgin olive oil

¼ cup red onion, minced

1 cup quinoa

¼ teaspoon turmeric or annatto, ground (for color)

2 cups water, vegetable, or low-sodium chicken stock

¼ cup red pepper, minced

¼ cup orange pepper, minced

¼ cup peas, frozen

3 scallions, minced

1 cup spinach, chopped

⅓ teaspoon sea salt

⅛ teaspoon cayenne pepper

1. Heat oil in a medium saucepot with a tight-fitting lid. Sauté onions and turmeric for 3–4 minutes until vegetables are softened. Add quinoa and continue to sauté for 1 minute longer until coated.

2. Add the water or stock. Bring to a boil. Lower to a simmer and cover tightly.

3. When all the liquid is absorbed and quinoa is tender, remove from flame. Cool 5 minutes and add the chopped vegetables. Combine well.

4. Season with salt and cayenne pepper.

EXCHANGES
1 STARCH
½ FAT

CALORIES 105
  CALORIES FROM FAT 20
TOTAL FAT 2.5 g
  SATURATED FAT 0.4 g
  TRANS FAT 0.0 g
CHOLESTEROL 0 mg
SODIUM 110 mg
POTASSIUM 195 mg
TOTAL CARBOHYDRATE 17 g
  DIETARY FIBER 3 g
  SUGARS 2 g
PROTEIN 4 g
PHOSPHORUS 120 mg

SNOW PEAS WITH POPPY SEEDS AND MATCHSTICK CARROTS

SERVES: 8   SERVING SIZE: ⅛ recipe

These ingredients form the perfect team of taste, color, and texture. Serve grilled shrimp or turkey breast steaks over these crunchy vegetables, which can also be served at room temperature.

2 teaspoons olive or canola oil

8 ounces (about 3 cups) sugar snap or snow peas

3 cups carrots, cut into matchstick size

1 tablespoon ginger root, freshly minced

1 teaspoon poppy seeds

¼ teaspoon sea salt

⅛ teaspoon ground black pepper

1. Heat oil in a large sauté pan over medium-high heat. Add the sugar snap or snow peas, carrots, ginger, and poppy seeds. Sauté for 3–4 minutes until tender-crisp. Season with salt and pepper.

EXCHANGES
1 VEGETABLE
½ FAT

CALORIES 40
  CALORIES FROM FAT 15
TOTAL FAT 1.5 g
  SATURATED FAT 0.2 g
  TRANS FAT 0.0 g
CHOLESTEROL 0 mg
SODIUM 105 mg
POTASSIUM 160 mg
TOTAL CARBOHYDRATE 6 g
  DIETARY FIBER 2 g
  SUGARS 3 g
PROTEIN 1 g
PHOSPHORUS 30 mg

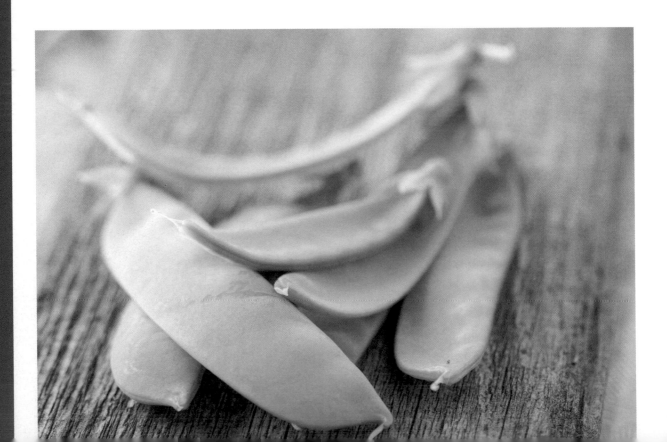

CRUNCHY CAJUN CABBAGE SLAW

SERVES: 12   **SERVING SIZE**: 1/12 recipe

Think of this as a power slaw with various cruciferous vegetables that taste delicious and don't even hint at their nutritional prowess.

DRESSING

- 1/2 cup low-fat mayonnaise
- 1/2 cup fat-free Greek yogurt
- 1 tablespoon Dijon-style mustard
- 3 tablespoons apple cider vinegar
- 2 tablespoons agave or honey
- 1 teaspoon sea or kosher salt
- 1 teaspoon blackening spice

SLAW VEGETABLES

- 5 cups green cabbage, thinly sliced
- 3 cups red cabbage, thinly sliced
- 4 kale or collard green leaves, heavy stem removed, thinly sliced
- 2 carrots, peeled and shredded
- 4 scallions, minced

1. Combine dressing ingredients in a large mixing bowl with a wire whisk.

2. Add vegetables and mix well. Allow to marinate for at least 1 hour before serving.

EXCHANGES
1/2 CARBOHYDRATE
1 VEGETABLE

CALORIES 55
  CALORIES FROM FAT 10
TOTAL FAT 1.0 g
  SATURATED FAT 0.1 g
  TRANS FAT 0.0 g
CHOLESTEROL 0 mg
SODIUM 335 mg
POTASSIUM 215 mg
TOTAL CARBOHYDRATE 10 g
  DIETARY FIBER 2 g
  SUGARS 6 g
PROTEIN 2 g
PHOSPHORUS 45 mg

SIDEKICKS

103

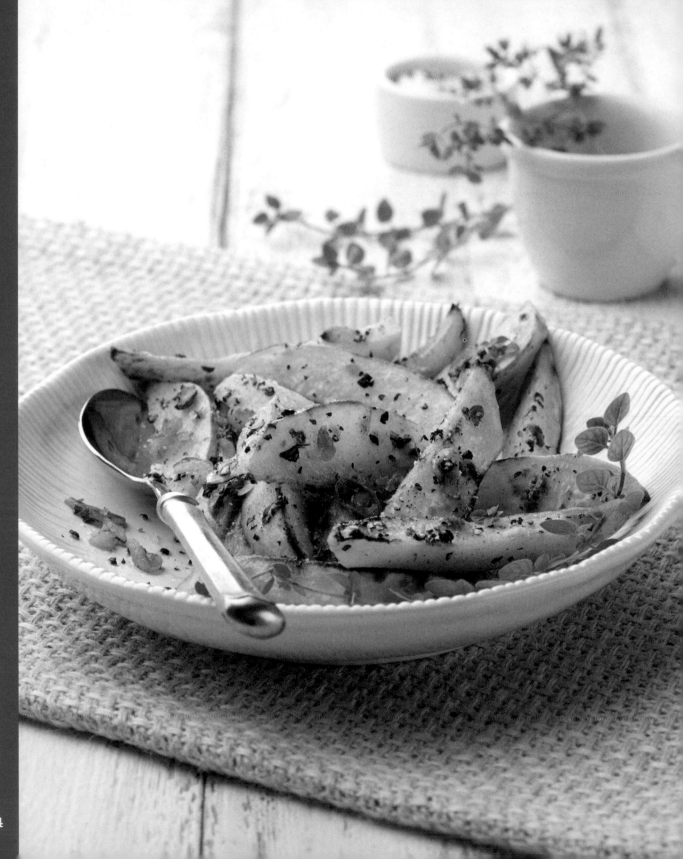

GREEK ROAST POTATOES WITH LEMON AND GARLIC

SERVES: 4   **SERVING SIZE**: 1/4 recipe

Authentic and served with almost every entrée in Greece, this dish is one of my favorite side dishes to serve with grilled meats, poultry, and seafood. Simple and tangy in flavor, it can be made ahead of time and is really good cold.

2 pounds all-purpose potatoes, peeled and cut into wedges

2 tablespoons extra virgin olive oil

1/3 cup lemon juice, fresh or bottled

3 cloves garlic, sliced thin

1 teaspoon oregano, dried (or 2 teaspoons fresh)

1/2 teaspoon turmeric

1 1/2 cups low-sodium vegetable or chicken stock

1/2 teaspoon kosher salt

1/4 teaspoon black pepper, ground

1. Peel and cut the potatoes, placing them in water while you do so. Preheat oven to 375°F.

2. Combine the drained potatoes, olive oil, lemon juice, garlic, oregano, and turmeric in a large mixing bowl and marinate for 10 minutes.

3. Place potatoes in a large roasting pan with marinade, stock, salt, and pepper. Roast uncovered for approximately 55 minutes, turning occasionally, until potatoes are tender and lightly browned.

EXCHANGES
2 STARCH
1 FAT

CALORIES 200
  CALORIES FROM FAT 65
TOTAL FAT 7.0 g
  SATURATED FAT 1.0 g
  TRANS FAT 0.0 g
CHOLESTEROL 0 mg
SODIUM 305 mg
POTASSIUM 765 mg
TOTAL CARBOHYDRATE 31 g
  DIETARY FIBER 4 g
  SUGARS 3 g
PROTEIN 4 g
PHOSPHORUS 125 mg

WILTED GARLIC AND POPPY SEED SPINACH

SERVES: 4   **SERVING SIZE**: ¼ recipe

So simple and so good, fresh spinach leaves with just a few ingredients—the perfect accompaniment for anything cooked on the grill.

1 tablespoon olive oil
3 cloves garlic, thinly sliced
2 pounds spinach leaves
¼ cup poppy seeds
Water as needed
Salt, to taste
Freshly ground black pepper, to taste

1. In a large nonstick skillet, heat oil over medium heat. Add garlic and let begin to brown lightly.

2. As soon as garlic browns, add spinach and stir well, adding a few drops of water to slow the browning process.

3. Sauté 2 minutes just until wilted, add the poppy seeds, and season with salt and pepper.

EXCHANGES
2 VEGETABLE
1½ FAT

CALORIES 130
  CALORIES FROM FAT 70
TOTAL FAT 8.0 g
  SATURATED FAT 1.0 g
  TRANS FAT 0.0 g
CHOLESTEROL 0 mg
SODIUM 180 mg
POTASSIUM 1335 mg
TOTAL CARBOHYDRATE 11 g
  DIETARY FIBER 7 g
  SUGARS 1 g
PROTEIN 8 g
PHOSPHORUS 190 mg

ARUGULA AND PARMESAN TOSS

SERVES: 4   **SERVING SIZE:** ¼ recipe

This arugula recipe is one of my favorite dishes. It's incredibly simple and, when served as a bed under any grilled chop or chicken breast, the dish gets elevated to a much higher place. The key here is using high-quality Parmesan (I recommend Reggiano or Padano) and high-quality extra virgin olive oil.

10 ounces arugula or baby arugula, well washed

 2 tablespoons extra virgin olive oil

⅓ cup shaved or shredded Parmesan cheese
    Juice of 1 lemon

½ teaspoon kosher salt

¼ teaspoon black pepper, ground (preferably freshly
    ground from a mill)

 1 tablespoon pine nuts, toasted (optional)

1. Combine all ingredients well, just before serving,
    and toss well. Place and serve immediately.

EXCHANGES
2 FAT

CALORIES 95
  CALORIES FROM FAT 70
TOTAL FAT 8.0 g
  SATURATED FAT 1.5 g
  TRANS FAT 0.0 g
CHOLESTEROL 0 mg
SODIUM 305 mg
POTASSIUM 280 mg
TOTAL CARBOHYDRATE 4 g
  DIETARY FIBER 1 g
  SUGARS 2 g
PROTEIN 3 g
PHOSPHORUS 60 mg

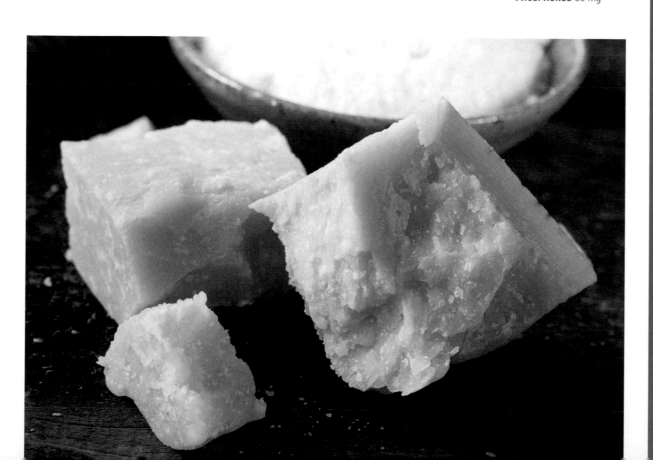

SIDEKICKS

CUBAN BLACK BEANS WITH CRACKED CUMIN AND LIME

SERVES: 3   **SERVING SIZE**: 1/3 recipe

Living in South Florida makes having a "go to" black bean recipe a necessity. I like them simmered and left whole, while some cooks purée them. These can be served as a side dish, as well as a burrito or quesadilla filling. I sometimes serve these over short-grain brown rice with chopped avocado, Greek yogurt, and shredded cheddar as my dinner on the nights I give my grill a break.

1 tablespoon canola oil
1 cup chopped red onion
1 cup canned chopped tomatoes
3/4 cup chopped green bell pepper
2 garlic cloves, minced
1 teaspoon crushed cumin seeds
1 (15-ounce) can black beans, undrained
1/4 cup minced fresh cilantro
1 tablespoon fresh lime juice

TOPPINGS (OPTIONAL)
Reduced-fat sour cream or fat-free Greek yogurt
Pickled jalapeños
Shredded low-fat cheddar cheese

1. Heat canola or olive oil in a large saucepot over medium heat. Add red onion, tomato, bell pepper, garlic, and cumin. Cook 4 minutes, stirring constantly, until tender.

2. Add beans, reduce heat to medium-low, and cook for 10 minutes.

3. Add cilantro and juice. Serve. Garnish with Greek yogurt, jalapeños, and shredded cheese, if desired.

EXCHANGES
1 STARCH
2 VEGETABLE
1/2 FAT

CALORIES 155
  CALORIES FROM FAT 35
TOTAL FAT 4.0 g
  SATURATED FAT 0.4 g
  TRANS FAT 0.0 g
CHOLESTEROL 0 mg
SODIUM 390 mg
POTASSIUM 575 mg
TOTAL CARBOHYDRATE 23 g
  DIETARY FIBER 6 g
  SUGARS 5 g
PROTEIN 7 g
PHOSPHORUS 150 mg

ORANGE CASHEW BASMATI RICE

SERVES: 9 **SERVING SIZE**: ¹/₄ cup

I've been making this dish for years because it has the whole package. It's beautiful to look at, tastes great, and goes with so many dishes. It's unusual because most rice pilafs are not made with orange juice in the base liquid. Toasting the cashews gives them extra flavor and aroma. I sometimes substitute dried unsweetened coconut for the cashews.

1 tablespoon canola or peanut oil

1 cup onion, chopped

¹/₂ teaspoon turmeric, ground

1¹/₂ cups basmati rice

¹/₂ cup orange juice

1 cup water or vegetable or low-sodium chicken stock

¹/₂ cup roasted cashews, chopped

¹/₂ cup unsweetened mandarin orange sections, drained

¹/₂ teaspoon kosher salt

¹/₄ teaspoon cayenne pepper

1 tablespoon butter (optional)

1. Heat oil in a 3-to-4 quart saucepot with a tight-fitting lid.

2. Add onion and turmeric and sauté for 2 minutes (just enough to color the onions). Add rice and stir well.

3. Add the orange juice and water and bring to a boil. Lower to a simmer and cover tightly. Cook for 15–18 minutes until rice is just cooked and liquid is absorbed.

4. Add the cashews, salt, pepper, and butter, if using. Fluff before serving with a spoon.

EXCHANGES
2 STARCH
¹/₂ FAT

CALORIES 180
  CALORIES FROM FAT 45
TOTAL FAT 5.0 g
  SATURATED FAT 0.9 g
  TRANS FAT 0.0 g
CHOLESTEROL 0 mg
SODIUM 155 mg
POTASSIUM 155 mg
TOTAL CARBOHYDRATE 30 g
  DIETARY FIBER 1 g
  SUGARS 4 g
PROTEIN 4 g
PHOSPHORUS 85 mg

WARM POTATO SALAD WITH BACON AND CARAMELIZED ONIONS

SERVES: 6   **SERVING SIZE**: 1/6 recipe

I learned how to make the authentic version of this warm potato salad in Germany when I was working there decades ago.

2 pounds all-purpose potatoes (waxy kind), peeled
2 slices bacon, chopped
1 cup onion, chopped
1/4 cup vinegar, white or apple cider
1 tablespoon Dijon-style mustard
1/4 cup water
1 tablespoon honey
1/2 teaspoon kosher salt
1/4 teaspoon black pepper, ground
1/4 cup parsley, chopped

1. Boil potatoes until tender, about 15–18 minutes. Drain, cool, and set aside on a plate. Cool slightly and slice 1/4-inch thick.

2. Heat a large saucepan over medium-high heat and add bacon. Continue to sauté until bacon begins to crisp. Add onions. Continue to sauté 2 minutes until onions soften. Add vinegar, mustard, water, and honey. Combine well.

3. Add sliced potatoes, salt, pepper, and parsley. Serve warm.

EXCHANGES
2 STARCH
1/2 FAT

CALORIES 170
  CALORIES FROM FAT 40
TOTAL FAT 4.5 g
  SATURATED FAT 1.7 g
  TRANS FAT 0.0 g
CHOLESTEROL 5 mg
SODIUM 280 mg
POTASSIUM 455 mg
TOTAL CARBOHYDRATE 29 g
  DIETARY FIBER 3 g
  SUGARS 5 g
PROTEIN 3 g
PHOSPHORUS 70 mg

GRILLED MARINATED PICKLED PEPPERS

SERVES: 8   **SERVING SIZE**: 1/8 recipe

This is a modern grilled version of my mom's pickled peppers. She used to make them using only the sun as a pickling agent. They would sit in a giant jar on the porch for exactly 3 days to pickle. This is a quick pickle version. I think of her every time I make them.

1 red pepper, seeded and cut into strips
1 green pepper, seeded and cut into strips
1 yellow pepper, seeded and cut into strips
1 red onion, sliced
1 jalapeño, split, seeds intact
1 tablespoon pickling spices, salt-free
1 1/2 cups cider vinegar
1/2 cup water
2 tablespoons sugar
3 whole sprigs dill, tarragon, or oregano (optional)

1. Stuff the peppers into a glass jar in an attractive way. You can alternate rows of color or even add other vegetables like carrots, radish, or asparagus.

2. Boil all the remaining ingredients and pour over the vegetables, making sure you press them down and they are submerged.

3. Cool at room temperature, then close and refrigerate. The next day they can be served.

EXCHANGES
1 VEGETABLE

CALORIES 30
  CALORIES FROM FAT 0
TOTAL FAT 0.0 g
  SATURATED FAT 0.0 g
  TRANS FAT 0.0 g
CHOLESTEROL 0 mg
SODIUM 0 mg
POTASSIUM 165 mg
TOTAL CARBOHYDRATE 6 g
  DIETARY FIBER 1 g
  SUGARS 4 g
PROTEIN 1 g
PHOSPHORUS 20 mg

AGAVE LIME ROASTED PEPITAS

SERVES: 6   **SERVING SIZE**: ¹⁄₆ recipe

Frozen plantains will save you time, but feel free to use fresh if you prefer. I eat these with everything and sometimes serve them as a dessert with dulce de leche ice cream or lemon sorbet.

3 cups frozen sliced plantains

¹⁄₃ cup unsalted pumpkin seed kernels

2 tablespoons agave, lightly heated

¹⁄₄ teaspoon salt

Cooking spray

2 tablespoons fresh lime juice

1. Preheat oven to 400°F.

2. Place plantains in a large saucepan. Add water to just cover. Bring to a boil. Cook 3–4 minutes or until barely tender. Drain and transfer to large bowl. Stir in pumpkin seeds (pepitas), agave, and salt.

3. Spread mixture on baking pan lined with foil and coated with cooking spray. Bake at 400°F for 15 minutes, turning once. Drizzle with lime juice.

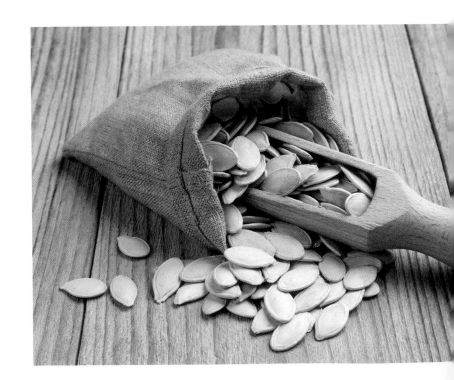

EXCHANGES
1¹⁄₂ STARCH
¹⁄₂ CARBOHYDRATE

CALORIES 150
  CALORIES FROM FAT 30
TOTAL FAT 3.5 g
  SATURATED FAT 0.6 g
  TRANS FAT 0.0 g
CHOLESTEROL 0 mg
SODIUM 105 mg
POTASSIUM 415 mg
TOTAL CARBOHYDRATE 31 g
  DIETARY FIBER 2 g
  SUGARS 16 g
PROTEIN 3 g
PHOSPHORUS 100 mg

BOBBY K'S SCALLOPED MUSHROOMS

SERVES: 6   **SERVING SIZE:** 1/6 recipe

The best way to make this easy recipe is with a multitude of mushroom varieties. I buy buttons, criminis, shiitakes, hedgehog, portabella, and a beautiful cinnamon-colored mushroom called a Hazel Dell. This dish makes a fine topping for any red meat or poultry.

1 tablespoon olive oil

1 large shallot, minced

2 cloves garlic, minced

1 pound assorted mushrooms, cleaned and sliced thick or in half depending on size

1/2 cup dry white wine, such as Chardonnay, Sauvignon Blanc, or a Dry Riesling

1/2 cup fat-free half-and-half cream

2 tablespoons fresh herbs, such as tarragon, parsley, basil (snipped with kitchen shears)

2 teaspoons butter, unsalted

1/2 teaspoon kosher salt

1/4 teaspoon crushed red chili flakes

1. Heat a large sauté pan over medium-high heat. Add oil and sauté the shallot and garlic for 30 seconds to soften and release their flavors.

2. Add the mushrooms and mix them into the sautéed shallot and garlic. Continue to sauté, only stirring occasionally until the mushrooms begin to color.

3. Continue to sauté, adding the wine and mixing well. Reduce the liquid in the pan and add the half-and-half. Continue to simmer for 2 minutes to thicken the pan juices.

4. Add the herbs, butter and salt, and chili flakes. Serve immediately.

EXCHANGES
1 VEGETABLE
1 FAT

CALORIES 75
  CALORIES FROM FAT 35
TOTAL FAT 4.0 g
  SATURATED FAT 1.3 g
  TRANS FAT 0.1 g
CHOLESTEROL 5 mg
SODIUM 180 mg
POTASSIUM 315 mg
TOTAL CARBOHYDRATE 6 g
  DIETARY FIBER 1 g
  SUGARS 2 g
PROTEIN 3 g
PHOSPHORUS 100 mg

GRILLED CREAMED CORN

SERVES: 6   **SERVING SIZE**: $1/6$ recipe

When you are grilling your dinner, throw the corn on afterwards for the next day's side dish. Corn can be grilled with the husk removed for a more charred flavor, or you can leave the husk on, which steams the corn and keeps it a bit juicier.

6 ears corn, grilled and cooled
2 teaspoons butter, unsalted
2 teaspoons flour
$1/4$ cup fat-free half-and-half
$1/4$ cup 2% milk
1 tablespoon parsley, minced
$1/2$ teaspoon sea or kosher salt
$1/4$ teaspoon black pepper, ground

1. Cut the grilled corn from the cob and set aside. The corn can be grilled up to three days prior to making this side dish.

2. Heat the butter in a saucepot over medium heat. Add the corn and sauté for 1 minute. Add the flour and continue to sauté for 30 seconds to combine.

3. Add the half-and-half and milk. Stir to combine well and simmer for 10 minutes until lightly thickened.

4. With an immersion blender or food processor, coarsely purée half the creamed corn. Add parsley. Season with salt and pepper.

EXCHANGES
$1^1/2$ STARCH
$1/2$ FAT

CALORIES 125
  CALORIES FROM FAT 25
TOTAL FAT 3.0 g
  SATURATED FAT 1.2 g
  TRANS FAT 0.0 g
CHOLESTEROL 5 mg
SODIUM 195 mg
POTASSIUM 265 mg
TOTAL CARBOHYDRATE 24 g
  DIETARY FIBER 3 g
  SUGARS 6 g
PROTEIN 4 g
PHOSPHORUS 105 mg

GRILLED KALE WITH ORANGE AND CRUSHED RED CHILI

SERVES: 4   **SERVING SIZE**: ¼ recipe

I discovered this recipe by accident and it's become a favorite. I prefer lacinato, also called dinosaur kale, because it holds up well to the grill and has a stronger flavor than the curly variety, but you can use any kale you like.

2 bunches curly green or lacinato kale (also called dinosaur kale)

2 tablespoons extra virgin olive oil

Juice of 2 oranges

½ teaspoon crushed red chili flakes

1 tablespoon low-sodium soy sauce

2 oranges, sliced ½ inch thick for a grilled garnish (optional)

1. In a large saucepot, bring 2 quarts of water to a boil.

2. Plunge the kale left tied in bunches into the water and blanch for 1 minute. Immediately remove the kale from the boiling water and place into ice cold water to "shock," or stop the cooking process. Drain well and set aside on a paper towel or clean kitchen towel to dry.

3. Combine the remaining ingredients, which will be used to baste the kale.

4. Preheat grill to medium high and place on grill grate. Cook as per directions for direct heat method.

5. Place the kale bunches, still tied together, on the grill, fanning out the leaves so they make contact with the grill pan. Baste with the liquid and continue to grill and baste, turning occasionally, until charred and cooked through, about 4–5 minutes total.

6. If using oranges, simply brush with the marinade and grill until marked in a crisscross fashion, then arrange around kale.

EXCHANGES
3 VEGETABLE
1 FAT

CALORIES 135
  CALORIES FROM FAT 55
TOTAL FAT 6.0 g
  SATURATED FAT 0.9 g
  TRANS FAT 0.0 g
CHOLESTEROL 0 mg
SODIUM 170 mg
POTASSIUM 645 mg
TOTAL CARBOHYDRATE 18 g
  DIETARY FIBER 5 g
  SUGARS 6 g
PROTEIN 5 g
PHOSPHORUS 80 mg

NEPALESE POTATOES

SERVES: 6   **SERVING SIZE**: ¹/₆ recipe

A universally loved side dish that goes well with all grilled items. These potatoes turn bright yellow during roasting and are pleasantly spicy. Even people who don't like curry adore these spuds!

2 pounds small red bliss potatoes, skin on, cut into wedges

2 tablespoons extra virgin olive oil

1 tablespoon curry powder

4 cloves garlic, minced

1 tablespoon minced fresh ginger root

2 jalapeño peppers, sliced thinly

1 teaspoon kosher or sea salt

Juice of 1 lemon

1. Place all ingredients in a large mixing bowl and set aside at room temperature for at least 15 minutes to 1 hour.

2. Preheat oven to 375°F.

3. Spread out potatoes evenly on a baking pan lined with parchment paper.

4. Roast, turning occasionally, for 50 minutes to an hour until cooked through and golden brown.

EXCHANGES
2 STARCH
¹/₂ FAT

CALORIES 165
  CALORIES FROM FAT 45
TOTAL FAT 5.0 g
  SATURATED FAT 0.7 g
  TRANS FAT 0.0 g
CHOLESTEROL 0 mg
SODIUM 330 mg
POTASSIUM 755 mg
TOTAL CARBOHYDRATE 27 g
  DIETARY FIBER 3 g
  SUGARS 3 g
PROTEIN 3 g
PHOSPHORUS 105 mg

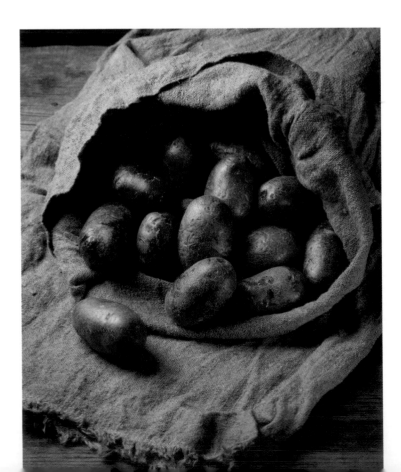

GRILLED HALLOUMI AND BAY LEAF SKEWERS

SERVES: 12   **SERVING SIZE**: 1 skewer

I originally had these little appetizer skewers in Sicily and have been making them ever since. You may use any good-quality Parmesan cheese, such as Grana Padano or Reggiano. If you prefer a less expensive cheese that also tastes great, try either Greek Halloumi or Latin queso blanco.

12 cubes Halloumi light cheese or Parmesan, cut in 1-inch cubes
24 pitted olives, kalamata if available
 1 tablespoon extra virgin olive oil
 1 tablespoon red wine vinegar or balsamic vinegar
 1 tablespoon oregano leaves, minced
12 each bay leaves, preferably fresh
     Wooden or metal skewers for grilling

1. Combine cheese, olives, olive oil, vinegar, and oregano in a small mixing bowl and marinate for at least 15 minutes or overnight.

2. Thread on skewers using 1 piece of cheese, 1 bay leaf, and 2 olives on each skewer.

3. Preheat grill to medium high and place on grill grate. Cook as per directions for direct heat method. Grill the skewers for 4–5 minutes until cheese begins to brown and soften.

EXCHANGES
1 FAT

CALORIES 50
  CALORIES FROM FAT 35
TOTAL FAT 4.0 g
  SATURATED FAT 1.3 g
  TRANS FAT 0.0 g
CHOLESTEROL 5 mg
SODIUM 130 mg
POTASSIUM 15 mg
TOTAL CARBOHYDRATE 1 g
  DIETARY FIBER 0 g
  SUGARS 0 g
PROTEIN 3 g
PHOSPHORUS 50 mg

GRILLED ASPARAGUS WITH TRUFFLE SALT AND PARMESAN

SERVES: 4   **SERVING SIZE**: ¼ recipe

Truffle salt can be found in most gourmet food stores and online. It has a rich earthy flavor that goes so well with good-quality olive oil and ground pepper. If you can't find truffle salt, use sea salt.

2 pounds asparagus
1 tablespoon extra virgin olive oil or melted unsalted butter
½ teaspoon truffle salt or sea salt
Freshly ground pepper
Parmesan cheese (optional)

1. Trim the last 2 inches of asparagus from ends and wash well. Place asparagus on a plate, drizzle the olive oil over, and rub into asparagus.

2. Preheat grill to medium high and place asparagus on grill grate. Grill the asparagus for 4–5 minutes until the spears begin to brown and soften. When tender, transfer to a serving dish and sprinkle with truffle salt and pepper. Scatter Parmesan cheese over, if desired, and serve.

EXCHANGES
1 VEGETABLE
½ FAT

CALORIES 55
  CALORIES FROM FAT 30
TOTAL FAT 3.5 g
  SATURATED FAT 0.5 g
  TRANS FAT 0.0 g
CHOLESTEROL 0 mg
SODIUM 290 mg
POTASSIUM 250 mg
TOTAL CARBOHYDRATE 5 g
  DIETARY FIBER 2 g
  SUGARS 1 g
PROTEIN 3 g
PHOSPHORUS 60 mg

BOILED FINGERLINGS WITH SMOKED SALT, DILL, AND GREEN ONION

SERVES: 4 **SERVING SIZE:** ¼ recipe

Nowadays you can find fingerlings, Peruvian purple potatoes, and lots of other kinds of potatoes in the produce section of your grocery or farmers' market. Smoked salt is also available in all gourmet food stores and online. It has a pleasant smoky flavor that goes well with all grilled items. If you can't find smoked salt, use sea salt.

1½ pounds fingerling potatoes, whole and unpeeled
1 tablespoon unsalted butter
¼ cup fresh dill, minced
1 bunch green onions or chives, minced
½ teaspoon smoked salt
Freshly ground pepper from a mill

1. Boil potatoes in salted water for 12–15 minutes until tender.

2. Drain and combine with remaining ingredients. Serve immediately.

EXCHANGES
2½ STARCH

CALORIES 175
 CALORIES FROM FAT 25
TOTAL FAT 3.0 g
 SATURATED FAT 1.9 g
 TRANS FAT 0.1 g
CHOLESTEROL 10 mg
SODIUM 305 mg
POTASSIUM 720 mg
TOTAL CARBOHYDRATE 35 g
 DIETARY FIBER 4 g
 SUGARS 2 g
PROTEIN 4 g
PHOSPHORUS 85 mg

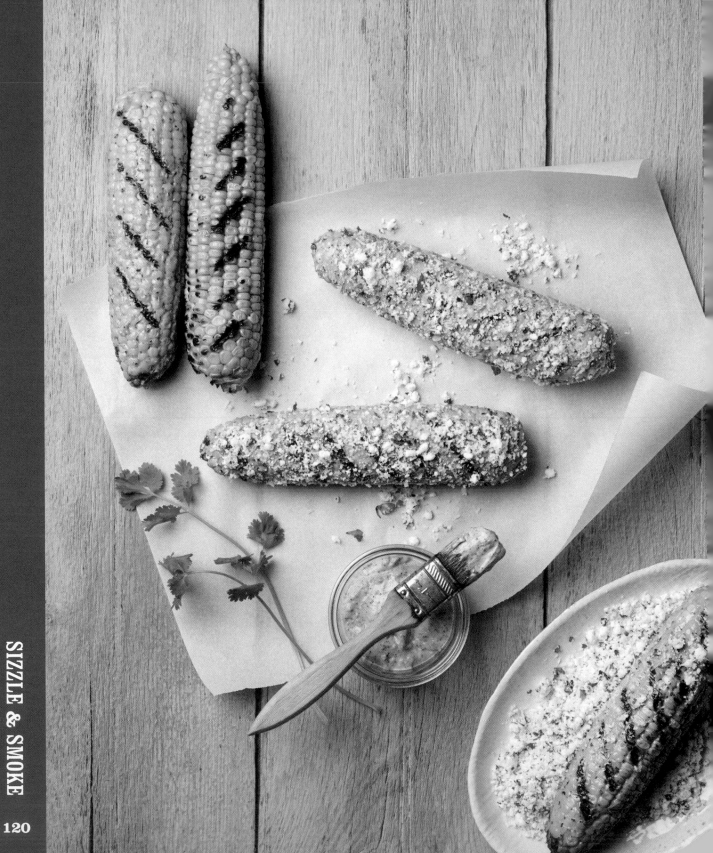

MEXICAN STREET CORN

SERVES: 6   **SERVING SIZE**: 1 ear

This is pretty much my favorite summer item to serve family and friends. When corn reaches peak season, I already have the rest of the recipe waiting in my fridge.

6 ears fresh corn, husks pulled down and cleaned but left attached

$1/2$ cup low-fat mayonnaise

1 tablespoon lemon juice

1 teaspoon dried oregano

$1/2$ teaspoon chili powder

$1/2$ teaspoon cumin

$1/3$ cup reduced-fat feta cheese, crumbled

$1/2$ cup Parmesan cheese, shredded

2 tablespoons fresh cilantro, minced

1. Boil or grill the corn until cooked through, about 5–6 minutes. If grilling, soak the corn and attached husks in water first so they don't burn.

2. Remove from the water or grill and trim off the husks, leaving about 2 inches to form a handle.

3. Combine the mayonnaise, lemon juice, oregano, chili powder, and cumin.

4. Spread the mayo mixture around the cooked corn evenly and place on a plate or large piece of parchment paper.

5. Combine the feta, Parmesan, and cilantro. Place on a large plate or piece of parchment paper and roll the corn into the cheese mixture. Pat the cheese onto the surface of the corn.

6. You may serve the corn at room temperature or place them in a 375°F oven for 10 minutes to heat through.

EXCHANGES
1$1/2$ STARCH
$1/2$ FAT

CALORIES 145
  CALORIES FROM FAT 40
TOTAL FAT 4.5 g
  SATURATED FAT 1.5 g
  TRANS FAT 0.0 g
CHOLESTEROL 5 mg
SODIUM 325 mg
POTASSIUM 255 mg
TOTAL CARBOHYDRATE 25 g
  DIETARY FIBER 3 g
  SUGARS 6 g
PROTEIN 7 g
PHOSPHORUS 135 mg

GRILLED AU GRATIN POTATOES

SERVES: 8   **SERVING SIZE**: ⅛ recipe

Who would have thought you could make au gratin potatoes in the grill? I love these potatoes as leftovers the next day, but there are rarely leftovers.

4 large baking potatoes, peeled and cut into small cubes

2 tablespoons extra virgin olive oil

2 cloves minced garlic

1 teaspoon smoked paprika

1 cup onions, thinly sliced

½ cup shredded low-fat cheddar or jack cheese (Cabot 50%)

½ cup fat-free half-and-half

1. Place the potatoes in a medium mixing bowl with the oil, garlic, paprika, onions, and cheese, and combine well.

2. Place the potatoes into 2 medium aluminum containers and pour half-and-half on top.

3. Preheat grill to medium-high heat and place pans on grill grate.

4. Close grill and cooked for 40–45 minutes, stirring occasionally, until potatoes are tender.

EXCHANGES
2 STARCH
1 FAT

CALORIES 195
  CALORIES FROM FAT 45
TOTAL FAT 5.0 g
  SATURATED FAT 1.4 g
  TRANS FAT 0.0 g
CHOLESTEROL 5 mg
SODIUM 65 mg
POTASSIUM 775 mg
TOTAL CARBOHYDRATE 33 g
  DIETARY FIBER 4 g
  SUGARS 3 g
PROTEIN 6 g
PHOSPHORUS 160 mg

MUSHROOM BARLEY WALNUT PILAF

SERVES: 4 SERVING SIZE: ¼ recipe

Pearled barley gives this pilaf a creamy taste, while the walnuts add pleasant crunch and character. Fresh-grated lemon peel creates a note of tart citrus. This dish is wonderful as a stuffing for chicken, pork, or fish. Feel free to use portabella, shiitake, or oyster mushrooms.

1 tablespoon olive or canola oil
1 onion, chopped (small)
1 large carrot, chopped
1 stalk celery, sliced
3 sprigs fresh thyme on the branch
1 cup pearled barley
2½ cups water or vegetable or chicken stock
1 cup mushrooms, sliced (can be a combination of any favorite varieties)
½ cup walnut pieces
1 teaspoon grated lemon peel
2 tablespoons chopped fresh parsley
Salt, to taste
Pepper, to taste

1. Heat oil in a 2½-quart saucepot over medium-high heat.

2. Add onion, carrot, celery, and thyme sprigs, and sauté for 2 minutes. Add pearled barley and continue to sauté to coat for 1 minute.

3. Add water or stock. Bring to a boil, lower to a simmer, and cover. Simmer for approximately 35–40 minutes. Add mushrooms, walnuts, lemon peel, and parsley. Season with salt and pepper. Allow to rest for 10 minutes for mushrooms to wilt and flavors to marry.

EXCHANGES
2 STARCH
1 VEGETABLE
2½ FAT

CALORIES 280
  CALORIES FROM FAT 125
TOTAL FAT 14.0 g
  SATURATED FAT 1.4 g
  TRANS FAT 0.0 g
CHOLESTEROL 0 mg
SODIUM 35 mg
POTASSIUM 355 mg
TOTAL CARBOHYDRATE 35 g
  DIETARY FIBER 6 g
  SUGARS 3 g
PROTEIN 7 g
PHOSPHORUS 165 mg

GREEK ORZO SALAD WITH PEAS, LEMON, AND KALAMATA OLIVES

SERVES: 6   **SERVING SIZE**: 1/6 recipe

You may use any small pasta shape for this salad. Add leftover grilled chicken breast or rotisserie chicken and turn this salad into an entrée.

8 ounces whole-wheat orzo, cooked al dente, drained and rinsed under cold water
1 cup English cucumber, diced 1/2 inch
1 cup tomato, chopped
1/2 cup red onion, chopped (half a medium onion)
1/4 cup kalamata olives, pitted and chopped
2 tablespoons dill, freshly minced
6 ounces reduced-fat feta cheese, crumbled
1/2 cup frozen peas, defrosted
1 tablespoon lemon juice, fresh
2 1/2 tablespoons extra virgin olive oil
1 teaspoon oregano, dried
1 heaping cup baby spinach leaves

1. Combine all ingredients except spinach leaves in a large bowl. Marinate at least one hour in refrigerator, covered, before serving. Add spinach leaves just before serving.

EXCHANGES
2 STARCH
1 VEGETABLE
2 FAT

CALORIES 260
  CALORIES FROM FAT 100
TOTAL FAT 11.0 g
  SATURATED FAT 2.5 g
  TRANS FAT 0.0 g
CHOLESTEROL 10 mg
SODIUM 350 mg
POTASSIUM 260 mg
TOTAL CARBOHYDRATE 34 g
  DIETARY FIBER 5 g
  SUGARS 3 g
PROTEIN 11 g
PHOSPHORUS 185 mg

QUICK BARBEQUE BEANS

SERVES: 8   **SERVING SIZE**: ⅛ recipe

Fast and furious with tremendous flavor, which tastes like you've stayed up all night simmering these beans. I like them cold as well. You can combine any variety of beans for this recipe. Bacon is an option but a mighty fine one.

- 2 teaspoons olive oil
- 1 cup onions, chopped
- 2 teaspoons smoked paprika
- 1 chipotle chili in adobo, minced
- 1 apple, cored, chopped
- ¼ cup barbeque sauce
- 2 tablespoons Dijon-style mustard
- 2 (16-ounce) cans pinto or cannellini beans
- 3 slices bacon, minced (optional)

1. Heat olive oil in a 2-quart saucepot over medium heat and add onions, smoked paprika, chipotle chili, and apple. Sauté for 2 minutes and add barbeque sauce, Dijon mustard, and beans. If adding bacon, then sauté with vegetables in this step.

2. Simmer for 15 minutes until flavors combine.

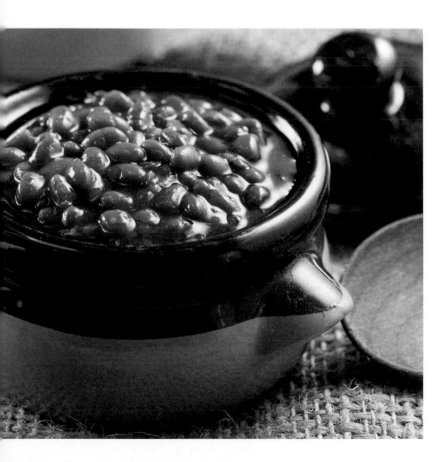

EXCHANGES
1 STARCH
1 CARBOHYDRATE

CALORIES 145
  CALORIES FROM FAT 20
TOTAL FAT 2.5 g
  SATURATED FAT 0.4 g
  TRANS FAT 0.0 g
CHOLESTEROL 0 mg
SODIUM 495 mg
POTASSIUM 365 mg
TOTAL CARBOHYDRATE 27 g
  DIETARY FIBER 6 g
  SUGARS 6 g
PROTEIN 6 g
PHOSPHORUS 120 mg

SOUTHERN-STYLE VEGETABLE CASSEROLE

SERVES: 10   **SERVING SIZE**: $^1/_{10}$ recipe

This is a much lighter version of a classic Deep South recipe served at many little barbeque joints.

Vegetable oil (for spraying pan)
1 small onion, sliced thin
1 green pepper, sliced thin
1 red pepper, sliced thin
2 medium zucchini, sliced thin lengthwise
2 medium yellow squash, sliced thin lengthwise
$^1/_2$ cup shredded reduced-fat sharp cheddar cheese
1 (8-ounce) container, fat-free sour cream or Greek yogurt
1 (10.75-ounce) can lower-fat cream of mushroom or celery soup
1 cup crushed saltines or Ritz crackers
1 tablespoon paprika
Salt, to paste
Pepper, to taste

1. Preheat the oven to 375°F.

2. Spray a 2-quart baking dish with vegetable oil and layer the vegetables over one another.

3. In a large bowl combine the cheese, sour cream, and soup. Mix well and spoon over the vegetables. Shake the casserole dish to distribute the sauce well.

4. In another small bowl, combine the crackers, paprika, salt, and pepper.

5. Sprinkle the crumb mixture evenly over the casserole and bake uncovered for 30 minutes until golden brown and crusty.

EXCHANGES
1 CARBOHYDRATE
1 VEGETABLE
$^1/_2$ FAT

CALORIES 110
  CALORIES FROM FAT 25
TOTAL FAT 3.0 g
  SATURATED FAT 1.1 g
  TRANS FAT 0.0 g
CHOLESTEROL 5 mg
SODIUM 250 mg
POTASSIUM 535 mg
TOTAL CARBOHYDRATE 17 g
  DIETARY FIBER 2 g
  SUGARS 5 g
PROTEIN 5 g
PHOSPHORUS 115 mg

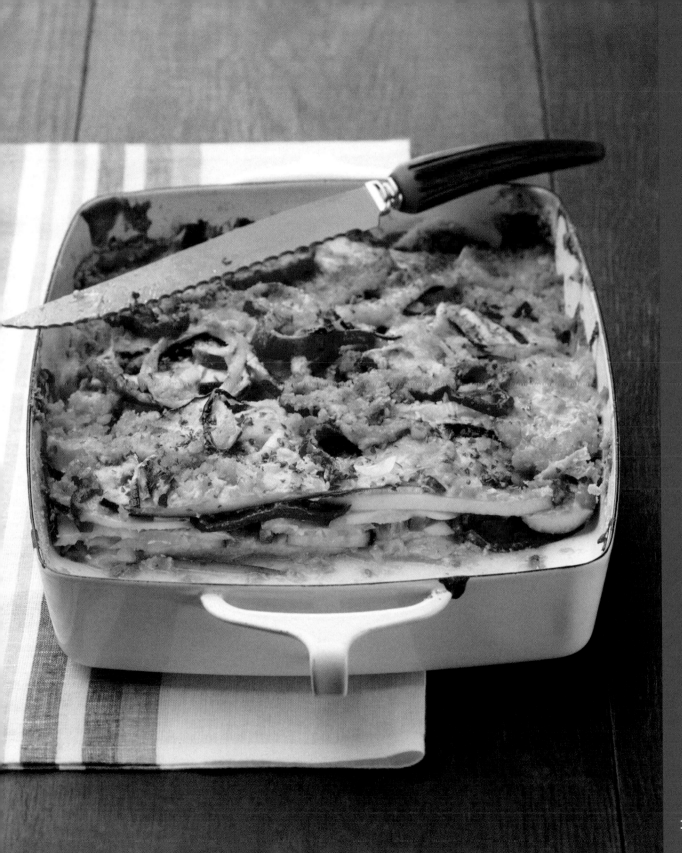

MAC N CHEESE SALAD

SERVES: 6   **SERVING SIZE**: ¹/₆ recipe

I always crave a great macaroni salad, potato salad, or slaw when I make grilled foods. This is one salad I always come back to. You can use a high-protein or whole-grain pasta instead of traditional elbow noodles if you prefer.

2 cups cooked elbow macaroni pasta

¹/₂ cup reduced-fat shredded cheese, such as cheddar, jack, or any combination

¹/₄ cup low-fat mayonnaise

1 tablespoon rice or cider vinegar

1 teaspoon Dijon-style mustard

1 cup rib celery, sliced

4 scallions, minced

¹/₂ cup carrot, peeled and grated

¹/₄ cup frozen green peas

¹/₄ cup parsley, minced

1. Combine all ingredients well in a large nonreactive mixing bowl. Make a day before so flavors meld with one another.

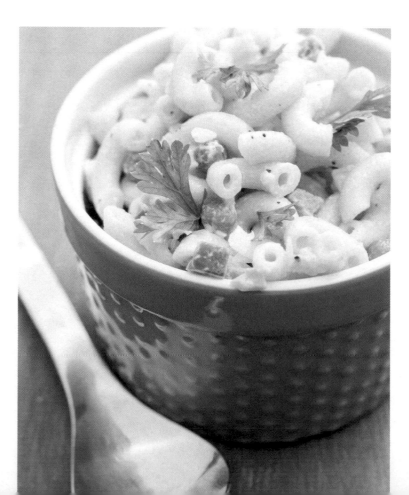

EXCHANGES
1 STARCH
¹/₂ FAT

CALORIES 125
  CALORIES FROM FAT 30
TOTAL FAT 3.5 g
  SATURATED FAT 1.4 g
  TRANS FAT 0.0 g
CHOLESTEROL 5 mg
SODIUM 215 mg
POTASSIUM 165 mg
TOTAL CARBOHYDRATE 19 g
  DIETARY FIBER 2 g
  SUGARS 2 g
PROTEIN 6 g
PHOSPHORUS 105 mg

QUINOA PILAF WITH APRICOTS, ALMONDS, AND PUMPKIN SEEDS

SERVES: 8   **SERVING SIZE**: ¹/₈ recipe

This recipe is a takeoff on the classic tabbouleh, which is cracked wheat with cucumbers and tomatoes. An Arabic friend explained that dried fruit and cracked wheat were the only ingredients that would survive a trip across the desert. It is loaded with flavor, fiber, and fruit. I make my version with high-protein quinoa as a replacement for cracked wheat.

1¹/₂ cups quinoa, raw
  3 cups water
¹/₂ cup dried apricots, chopped
¹/₄ cup dried dates, chopped
  1 cup cooked chickpeas
  1 cup chopped fresh mint
  1 cup chopped fresh parsley
¹/₄ cup sliced almonds
  2 tablespoons pumpkin seeds
¹/₄ cup lemon juice
¹/₄ cup extra virgin olive oil
¹/₂ teaspoon black pepper
¹/₂ teaspoon salt

1. Cook quinoa with a tight-fitting lid. Allow to rest for an hour to cool and place in a large bowl and fluff with a large spoon.

2. Add all the remaining ingredients and combine. Chill for 1 hour and serve alone or over salad greens.

EXCHANGES
2 STARCH
¹/₂ FRUIT
2 FAT

CALORIES 290
  CALORIES FROM FAT 110
TOTAL FAT 12.0 g
  SATURATED FAT 1.6 g
  TRANS FAT 0.0 g
CHOLESTEROL 0 mg
SODIUM 165 mg
POTASSIUM 505 mg
TOTAL CARBOHYDRATE 40 g
  DIETARY FIBER 7 g
  SUGARS 12 g
PROTEIN 9 g
PHOSPHORUS 250 mg

SIDEKICKS

SPINACH LIME CILANTRO ORZO

SERVES: 4 **SERVING SIZE**: ¼ recipe

Pearl-shaped orzo pasta gently takes on the flavor of any ingredient it is mixed with. In this case, sweet caramelized onions, leaf spinach, and garlic infuse each grain of pasta with pure taste.

8 ounces orzo pasta, uncooked
2 teaspoons olive oil
1 cup chopped onion
2 cups frozen chopped spinach
⅓ cup chopped fresh cilantro leaves
⅓ cup minced green onion
2 tablespoons fresh lime juice
½ teaspoon salt
¼ teaspoon cayenne pepper

1. Cook orzo al dente according to directions on bag or box. Drain and rinse well. Set aside in a bowl.

2. Heat oil in a large skillet over medium heat. Add onion and sauté for 3–4 minutes until lightly browned. Add the spinach and continue to sauté for another minute. Add the cooked orzo and all remaining ingredients and combine well.

EXCHANGES
2½ STARCH
2 VEGETABLE
½ FAT

CALORIES 255
  CALORIES FROM FAT 30
TOTAL FAT 3.5 g
  SATURATED FAT 0.5 g
  TRANS FAT 0.0 g
CHOLESTEROL 0 mg
SODIUM 355 mg
POTASSIUM 410 mg
TOTAL CARBOHYDRATE 47 g
  DIETARY FIBER 5 g
  SUGARS 7 g
PROTEIN 10 g
PHOSPHORUS 130 mg

SUMMER STRAWBERRY SLAW WITH CHIA SEEDS AND FLAX

SERVES: 16   **SERVING SIZE**: ¹/₁₆ recipe

Refreshing, colorful, vibrant, and full of vitamins and antioxidants, consider this a power slaw that is great served as a side dish or as a topping for tacos and sandwiches. You may add other berries as well. This can be also be made by omitting the yogurt. Chia and flax seeds add crunch and powerful antioxidants.

1 head green cabbage, thinly sliced

¹/₂ head red cabbage, thinly sliced

4 large carrots, grated or julienned

2 tablespoons honey or agave

¹/₂ cup raspberry vinegar

¹/₂ teaspoon kosher salt

¹/₄ teaspoon white pepper

¹/₂ teaspoon lemon zest

¹/₄ cup sliced almonds

2 tablespoons chia seeds

1 tablespoon flax seeds

1 cup fat-free honey or vanilla Greek yogurt

2 pints strawberries, sliced

1. Combine all ingredients in a large mixing bowl, gently mixing in strawberries last. Allow the slaw to marinate for 15 minutes before serving.

EXCHANGES
1¹/₂ CARBOHYDRATE

CALORIES 100
  CALORIES FROM FAT 15
TOTAL FAT 1.5 g
  SATURATED FAT 0.2 g
  TRANS FAT 0.0 g
CHOLESTEROL 0 mg
SODIUM 105 mg
POTASSIUM 395 mg
TOTAL CARBOHYDRATE 20 g
  DIETARY FIBER 5 g
  SUGARS 13 g
PROTEIN 4 g
PHOSPHORUS 90 mg

SIDEKICKS

SMOKY GAZPACHO SALAD

SERVES: 6   **SERVING SIZE**: 1/6 recipe

Although this salad can be made year round, it's truly best in summer or when you can get freshly picked produce. Try using different cucumber varieties like little Kirbys and English cucumbers. Try using heirloom tomatoes for color and diverse flavor. For an extra flavor pop, toast the almonds lightly in a 325°F oven for 5 minutes until golden brown.

- 2 cups peeled, diced cucumber (if the seeds are large, remove)
- 1/2 cup red bell pepper, diced
- 1/2 cup yellow pepper, diced
- 2 cups ripe tomatoes, diced
- 1/4 cup red onion, minced
- 1/2 cup basil, minced
- 1/4 cup extra virgin olive oil
- 1/4 cup red wine vinegar
- 2 teaspoons smoked Spanish paprika
- 1 clove garlic, minced
- 1/2 teaspoon kosher or sea salt
- 1/4 cup sliced almonds

1. Combine all ingredients well and allow to marinate for 20 minutes before serving.

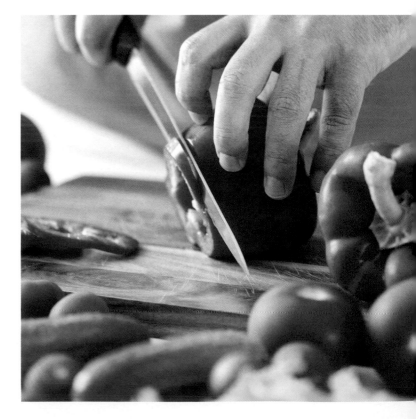

EXCHANGES
1 VEGETABLE
2 FAT

CALORIES 135
  CALORIES FROM FAT 100
TOTAL FAT 11.0 g
  SATURATED FAT 1.4 g
  TRANS FAT 0.0 g
CHOLESTEROL 0 mg
SODIUM 160 mg
POTASSIUM 330 mg
TOTAL CARBOHYDRATE 7 g
  DIETARY FIBER 2 g
  SUGARS 4 g
PROTEIN 2 g
PHOSPHORUS 55 mg

"ENLIGHTENED" FRIED RICE

SERVES: 10   **SERVING SIZE**: $^1/_{10}$ recipe

I make this dish with any kind of grain that I have in my pantry. I also combine cooked grains like brown rice and quinoa. Go ahead and add leftover grilled meat or vegetables to this dish to stretch it even further.

4 cups brown rice, cooked
1 tablespoon canola oil
2 teaspoons sesame oil
1 cup onion, diced
$^1/_2$ cup celery, diced
$^1/_2$ cup carrot, diced
$^1/_4$ cup red pepper, diced
2 cloves garlic, minced
2 teaspoons ginger, minced
$^1/_2$ teaspoon red pepper flakes
$^1/_4$ cup scallion, sliced
2 tablespoons reduced-sodium soy sauce

1. Cook rice according to directions. Heat canola and sesame oil in a large nonstick sauté pan. Sauté onion, celery, carrot, pepper, garlic, ginger, and red pepper flakes over medium heat for 2 minutes until slightly softened.

2. Add cooked rice, scallions, and soy sauce to the pan and continue to sauté until heated through.

EXCHANGES
1 STARCH
1 VEGETABLE
$^1/_2$ FAT

CALORIES 125
  CALORIES FROM FAT 25
TOTAL FAT 3.0 g
  SATURATED FAT 0.4 g
  TRANS FAT 0.0 g
CHOLESTEROL 0 mg
SODIUM 125 mg
POTASSIUM 120 mg
TOTAL CARBOHYDRATE 21 g
  DIETARY FIBER 2 g
  SUGARS 2 g
PROTEIN 3 g
PHOSPHORUS 80 mg

SIDEKICKS

CHAPTER 5
Desserts

I'm not a big dessert guy and never had a sweet tooth. I think that became more pronounced when I was diagnosed with prediabetes. I was just afraid to eat any sugar, knowing that it probably wasn't good for me. I pragmatically decided to use fresh fruit and alternative natural sweeteners as my dessert mantra. I also suggest relying on fresh, seasonal fruits, depending on where you live.

The one exception to this is the Dark Chocolate Poblano Smore's (page 146), which are truly delicious and very unique because they contain chocolate and spicy chipotle chilies. This recipe came to me when I was in a large test kitchen and several of my co-workers were crowded around a grill on a break. They were concocting their family favorite treat, melting marshmallows and chocolate together with spicy smoked chili peppers on graham crackers. Sometimes great recipes come to me in the weirdest ways. The Peach Tapioca Pudding (page 147) is another example of that kitchen accident that turns out to be a winner. I was in Georgia during peak peach season, making what I thought would be a peach sauce. I had no cornstarch or arrowroot, so I used tapioca powder to thicken the sauce lightly. I put it in the refrigerator to cool overnight, and the next day I had pudding instead. Delicious accidental peach pudding!

I always loved candy apples as a kid. I think you'll love the Cinnamon Ginger Apples (page 139). They are a grown-up candied apple dessert that brings me back to the days when life was carefree, before deadlines. The reality is that any fruit can be grilled and topped with nuts, seeds, or some kind of spice to enhance its natural flavor. Go ahead and experiment and have fun with your fruit on the grill.

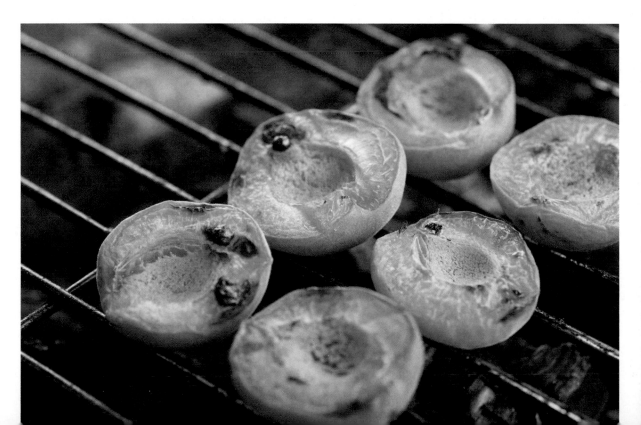

CINNAMON MAPLE GRILLED PEACHES

SERVES: 4   **SERVING SIZE**: 1 peach

I can't really find words for the flavor and mouth feel of this simple dessert. Serving them warm over the frozen ice cream is key. Garnish with fresh mint leaves and you can dress this dessert up nicely.

4 peaches or nectarines, still firm but ripe
   Juice of 1 lemon
¹/₂ teaspoon cinnamon
¹/₈ teaspoon nutmeg
1 tablespoon maple syrup

1. Preheat grill to medium high. Cook for 3–4 minutes, turning once, until golden brown on the outside, and just warmed through inside.

EXCHANGES
1 FRUIT

CALORIES 75
  CALORIES FROM FAT 0
TOTAL FAT 0.0 g
  SATURATED FAT 0.1 g
  TRANS FAT 0.0 g
CHOLESTEROL 0 mg
SODIUM 0 mg
POTASSIUM 305 mg
TOTAL CARBOHYDRATE 18 g
  DIETARY FIBER 2 g
  SUGARS 16 g
PROTEIN 1 g
PHOSPHORUS 30 mg

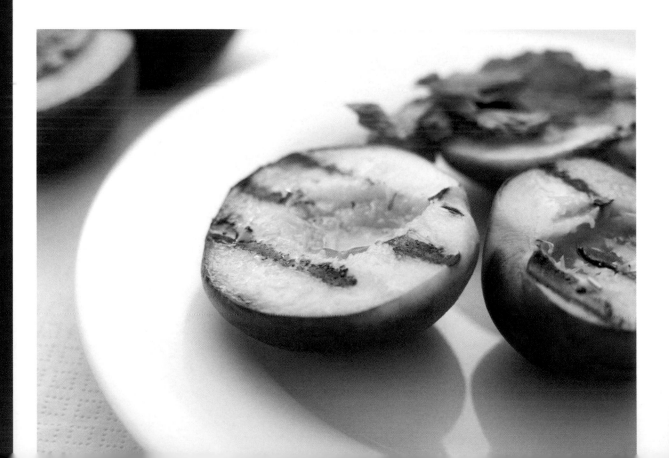

GRILLED PINEAPPLE STEAKS WITH RUM AND BLACK PEPPER YOGURT CREMA

SERVES: 4 **SERVING SIZE**: ¼ recipe

This is a really unusual, but easy, dessert. The tart pineapple and cooling crema is spiked with a bit of pepper and is a wonderful way to finish a meal.

- 4 (1-inch thick) rounds of fresh pineapple, core removed
- 2 tablespoons dark rum
- 1 teaspoon sesame seeds, brown, black, or a combination
- 1 tablespoon agave syrup
- ½ cup Greek fat-free yogurt, plain or vanilla
- ½ teaspoon grated lime zest
- ¼ teaspoon freshly milled black pepper

1. Combine pineapple with rum, sesame seeds, and agave for 15 minutes

2. Preheat grill to medium high. Cook as per directions for direct heat method for 3–4 minutes, turning once until golden brown on the outside, just warmed through inside. Set aside.

3. Make crema by combining the yogurt, lime zest, and black pepper.

4. Serve the grilled pineapple with crema over the top.

EXCHANGES
1 FRUIT
½ CARBOHYDRATE

CALORIES 105
 CALORIES FROM FAT 5
TOTAL FAT 0.5 g
 SATURATED FAT 0.1 g
 TRANS FAT 0.0 g
CHOLESTEROL 0 mg
SODIUM 15 mg
POTASSIUM 160 mg
TOTAL CARBOHYDRATE 20 g
 DIETARY FIBER 2 g
 SUGARS 16 g
PROTEIN 4 g
PHOSPHORUS 50 mg

DESSERTS

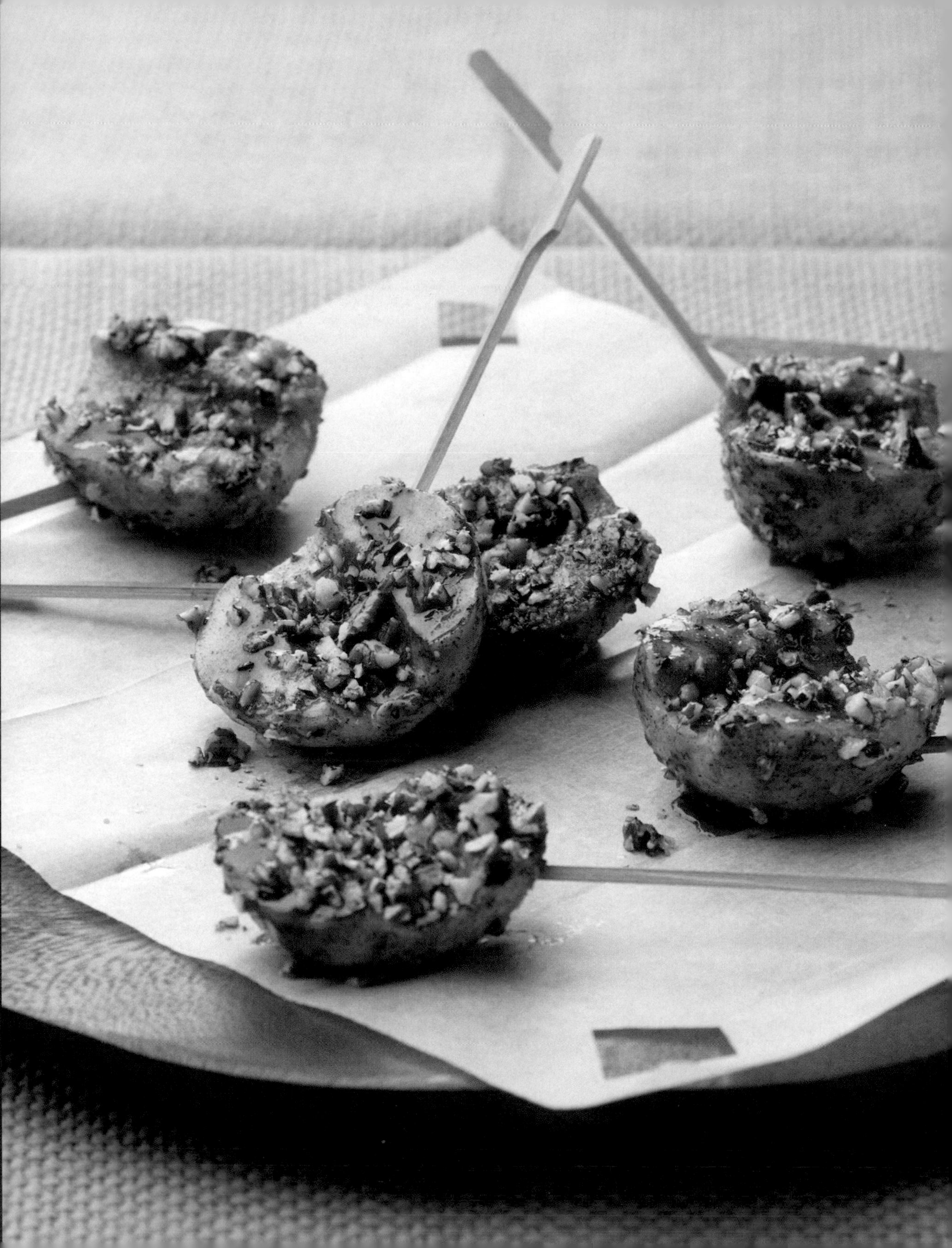

CINNAMON GINGER APPLE ON A STICK

SERVES: 6   **SERVING SIZE**: ¹/₂ apple

A novel approach to dessert. The crushed nuts add crunch and eye appeal. You can also cut the apples in quarters and place a few different varieties on each stick.

- 3 apples (Granny Smith, Fuji, Rome, or Gala), peeled, halved, and core removed
- Juice of 1 lemon
- 1 tablespoon minced fresh ginger root
- ¹/₂ teaspoon cinnamon
- 1 tablespoon honey
- ¹/₄ cup crushed walnuts or pecans
- 6 wooden or metal skewers

1. Marinate apple halves in all ingredients except walnuts.

2. Preheat grill to medium high. Cook as per directions for direct heat method (page 3) for 5–6 minutes, turning once until golden brown on the outside and just warmed through on the inside.

3. Remove apples from the grill, cool for a few minutes, and roll in crushed walnuts. Press gently.

4. Place a skewer in each apple half and serve.

EXCHANGES
1 FRUIT
¹/₂ FAT

CALORIES 75
  CALORIES FROM FAT 30
TOTAL FAT 3.5 g
  SATURATED FAT 0.3 g
  TRANS FAT 0.0 g
CHOLESTEROL 0 mg
SODIUM 0 mg
POTASSIUM 95 mg
TOTAL CARBOHYDRATE 13 g
  DIETARY FIBER 1 g
  SUGARS 10 g
PROTEIN 1 g
PHOSPHORUS 25 mg

GRILLED PEARS WITH GIN AND ALMONDS

SERVES: 4   **SERVING SIZE:** 1 pear

Use firm pears that are not quite ripe for this recipe. The aromatic gin pairs perfectly with the flavor of pears. Almonds add a welcome crunch.

4 pears (Bartlett, Anjou, or Bosc) halved, cored, and unpeeled

1 tablespoon butter blend, melted

1 tablespoon gin

2 teaspoons agave, or amber or maple syrup

1/2 teaspoon vanilla

   Juice of 1 lemon

1/4 cup almonds, sliced

1. Combine all of the ingredients, except almonds, in a medium bowl and put into a large, tightly sealed plastic bag. Marinate pear halves at least 15 minutes at room temperature.

2. Preheat grill to medium high and place on grill grate. Cook as per directions for direct heat method. Grill, turning occasionally, for 5–6 minutes until pears are marked well and tender.

3. Place almonds on a plate and roll grilled pears through the almonds, pressing gently to coat.

EXCHANGES
2 FRUIT
1 FAT

CALORIES 180
  CALORIES FROM FAT 55
TOTAL FAT 6.0 g
  SATURATED FAT 1.3 g
  TRANS FAT 0.0 g
CHOLESTEROL 5 mg
SODIUM 25 mg
POTASSIUM 260 mg
TOTAL CARBOHYDRATE 32 g
  DIETARY FIBER 6 g
  SUGARS 20 g
PROTEIN 2 g
PHOSPHORUS 50 mg

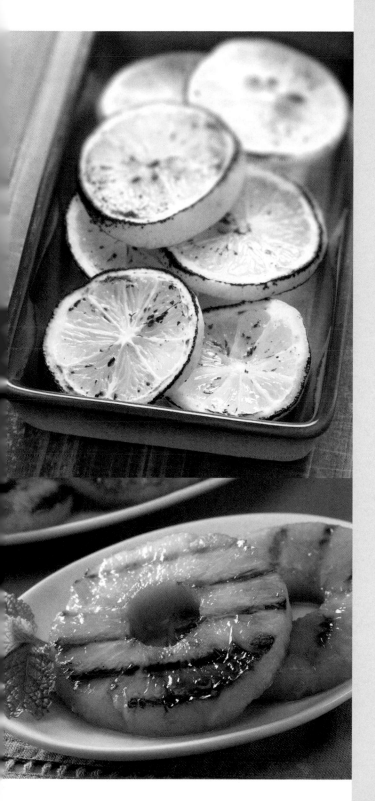

GRILLING FRUIT

Grilling fruit takes just as much savvy as poultry, seafood, or red meat. Most fruits contain large amounts of moisture, which makes browning them a bit of a challenge. Here are a few grilled fruit primers to keep in mind when making your meal:

- PICK FRUIT THAT IS JUST BARELY RIPE | the high heat of the grill will intensify the fresh fruit flavor and you won't have to worry about the fruit falling apart on the grill.

- GRILL FRUIT WITH THE SKIN ON | this will help the fruit keep its delicate character.

- USE A GRILL BASKET OR SKEWERS | preferably nonstick, as it will be easier to pull cooked fruit from grill.

- BASTE WITH A NEUTRAL OIL OR MELTED BUTTER | this will flavor the fruit and prevent it from sticking to the grill as well. Neutral oils such as canola, peanut, or safflower are best. Olive oils are pretty strong in flavor and will conceal the natural flavor of the fruit.

- SPRINKLE THE FRUIT WITH SWEETENER THE LAST FEW MINUTES OF GRILLING | you can use any sweetener you choose. It will caramelize in just a matter of seconds, so watch it to make sure it doesn't burn.

GRILLED BANANAS FOSTER

SERVES: 4   **SERVING SIZE**: 1/4 recipe

What a way to cap off a meal. This is a much lighter version of the classic Bananas Foster. You can make it with pears, apples, or any seasonal fruit. There are a few companies that make a decent sugar-free caramel sauce, but feel free to leave it out. Serve over sugar-free ice cream or Greek fat-free yogurt in a parfait glass and top with walnuts.

3 bananas, barely ripe, peeled

2 teaspoons Smart Balance butter substitute or butter

2 tablespoons Splenda light brown sugar mixture

2 tablespoons sugar-free caramel sauce

1/8 teaspoon cinnamon

1 tablespoon lemon juice

1 teaspoon vanilla extract

1/4 cup rum or Grand Marnier

1/4 cup chopped walnuts

1. Preheat grill to medium high and place bananas on grill grate. Cook as per directions for direct heat method. Grill for 3–5 minutes until slightly softened.

2. Heat butter substitute in a nonstick sauté pan over medium-high heat.

3. Add Splenda brown sugar mix, caramel sauce, cinnamon, lemon juice, vanilla, and rum or liqueur. Bring to a simmer and cook 4 minutes until sauce melts.

4. Slice grilled bananas and add to sauce. Add walnuts to the sauce.

EXCHANGES
2 1/2 CARBOHYDRATE
1 FAT

CALORIES 220
  CALORIES FROM FAT 65
TOTAL FAT 7.0 g
  SATURATED FAT 1.0 g
  TRANS FAT 0.0 g
CHOLESTEROL 0 mg
SODIUM 35 mg
POTASSIUM 395 mg
TOTAL CARBOHYDRATE 35 g
  DIETARY FIBER 3 g
  SUGARS 15 g
PROTEIN 2 g
PHOSPHORUS 50 mg

CITRUS POLENTA CAKE WITH DRIED FIGS, PISTACHIOS, AND OLIVE OIL

SERVES: 8   **SERVING SIZE:** ⅛ recipe

The first time I had this dessert was in Sicily. I had never really heard of polenta cake, but have been making it ever since. You can add any kind of dried fruit or nuts to this cake.

4 egg yolks
½ cup Splenda brown sugar baking blend
  Juice and zest of 1 orange
  Juice and zest of 1 lemon
2 cups 2% milk
¼ cup extra virgin olive oil
½ cup plus 1 tablespoon coarse cornmeal
½ teaspoon salt
¼ cup dried figs, chopped
¼ cup shelled pistachios, chopped
1 teaspoon fennel or anise seeds, crushed
  Vegetable oil for spraying baking pan

1. Preheat oven to 350°F.

2. Beat the egg yolks, Splenda mix, orange and lemon zest and juice in a mixing bowl and set aside.

3. Gently heat the milk and olive oil in a saucepan over medium heat. Slowly add the warmed milk to the egg yolks and return this mixture to low heat. Gradually add the cornmeal to the eggs and continue to stir until it almost boils.

4. Add the salt, figs, pistachios, and fennel seed to the mixture and pour into a small 8-inch baking pan sprayed with vegetable oil.

5. Bake uncovered for 35–40 minutes until baked through and the edges around the pan start to separate from sides. Remove from pan and cool for 15 minutes before serving.

EXCHANGES
2 CARBOHYDRATE
2 FAT

CALORIES 230
  CALORIES FROM FAT 100
TOTAL FAT 11.0 g
  SATURATED FAT 2.0 g
  TRANS FAT 0.0 g
CHOLESTEROL 90 mg
SODIUM 180 mg
POTASSIUM 235 mg
TOTAL CARBOHYDRATE 28 g
  DIETARY FIBER 1 g
  SUGARS 12 g
PROTEIN 5 g
PHOSPHORUS 130 mg

GRILLED ANGEL FOOD CAKE WITH MELTED BERRIES

SERVES: 8 **SERVING SIZE:** 1 slice

3 cups mixed berries, such as strawberries, blueberries, blackberries, and raspberries

1 teaspoon Splenda

1 tablespoon maple syrup

1/4 teaspoon cardamom, ground

12 teaspoons balsamic vinegar

1 8 ounce unfrosted angel food cake, cut into eight, 1-inch-thick slices

Vegetable oil (for spraying grill)

1. Line a medium bowl with a large piece of aluminum foil, pressing the foil into the sides of the bowl well.

2. Add the berries, Splenda, maple syrup, cardamom, and balsamic vinegar over all.

3. Wrap the foil up, forming a package, and twist the top so the liquid doesn't escape.

4. Preheat the grill over medium-high heat and place the berry package on the grill for the direct heat method (page 3).

5. Grill for 5–6 minutes, turning and shaking the package occasionally. Spray the cake slices lightly with vegetable oil to prevent sticking and add the cake slices to the grill to mark. Grill gently for 2–3 minutes, place on a serving dish and pour the melted berries over the cake.

6. If desired, serve with sugar-free whipped cream or low- or no-fat Greek yogurt.

EXCHANGES
2 CARBOHYDRATE

CALORIES 110
  CALORIES FROM FAT 0
TOTAL FAT 0.0 g
  SATURATED FAT 0.0 g
  TRANS FAT 0.0 g
CHOLESTEROL 0 mg
SODIUM 145 mg
POTASSIUM 125 mg
TOTAL CARBOHYDRATE 26 g
  DIETARY FIBER 2 g
  SUGARS 15 g
PROTEIN 2 g
PHOSPHORUS 80 mg

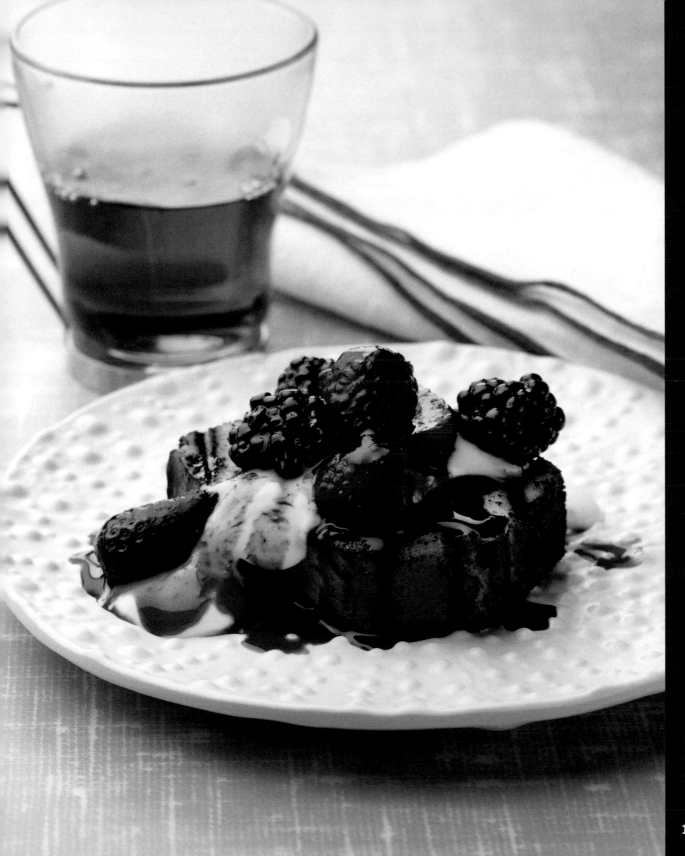

DARK CHOCOLATE POBLANO S'MORES

SERVES: 8   **SERVING SIZE**: ⅛ recipe

As a chef, throughout the country I work with some amazing cooks from all over Mexico. One day business was a bit slow and one of the cooks was making his family favorite treats for the staff. They blew me away and are quite unique. I think it's the spicy, sweet flavor that got me. If you don't feel like firing up the grill, you may broil the peppers until charred, or place them on a range-top heating element until black and charred before peeling.

- 2 medium-size poblano chili peppers
- 8 graham cracker sheets
- 2 ripe (but not overripe) bananas, peeled and sliced lengthwise ½-inch thick
- 1 (2.3-ounce) unsweetened dark chocolate (or chocolate of choice) bar, separated into squares or broken into pieces
- 8 marshmallows, sliced in half horizontally

1. Lightly oil the poblano peppers. Preheat grill to medium high and place peppers on grill grate. Cook as per directions for direct heat method (page 3) for 5–6 minutes until charred and tender. Set aside on a plate and cover with a clean kitchen towel. Cool.

2. Peel chilies and remove seeds and stems. Cut each pepper in half lengthwise and set aside on a paper towel to dry.

3. Place 4 graham crackers on a work surface. Place a half chili on each. Divide banana slices over chilies. Divide chocolate squares over bananas. Divide marshmallow rounds over the chocolate. Top with another graham cracker.

4. Place on a plate and microwave on high 1½ minutes until chocolate and marshmallows melt.

EXCHANGES
2 CARBOHYDRATE
½ FAT

CALORIES 160
  CALORIES FROM FAT 35
TOTAL FAT 4.0 g
  SATURATED FAT 1.8 g
  TRANS FAT 0.0 g
CHOLESTEROL 0 mg
SODIUM 95 mg
POTASSIUM 230 mg
TOTAL CARBOHYDRATE 30 g
  DIETARY FIBER 2 g
  SUGARS 17 g
PROTEIN 2 g
PHOSPHORUS 45 mg

PEACH TAPIOCA PUDDING

SERVES: 6   **SERVING SIZE**: ¹/₆ recipe

I discovered this purely by accident. I was making a fresh peach dessert sauce for a dinner party in Georgia. While the fresh peaches were simmering away, I realized that I had tapioca, but no cornstarch. Not only did it work well as a sauce, but when it cooled, the tapioca formed an incredible pudding.

8 fresh ripe peaches, sliced ¹/₂-inch thick
1 cup water or almond milk or 2% milk
3 tablespoons Splenda brown sugar blend
3 cinnamon sticks, whole
6 cloves
2 cardamom buds
1 tablespoon lemon zest
¹/₂ cup quick-cooking tapioca

1. Put all ingredients except tapioca in a saucepot and bring to a boil. Lower to a simmer and cook for 7–8 minutes until peaches melt.

2. Add tapioca and bring back to a boil. Simmer 3 minutes.

3. Eat warm over ice cream or frozen yogurt, or chill overnight in a glass container until it sets up into a pudding.

EXCHANGES
2¹/₂ CARBOHYDRATE

CALORIES 150
  CALORIES FROM FAT 0
TOTAL FAT 0.0 g
  SATURATED FAT 0.0 g
  TRANS FAT 0.0 g
CHOLESTEROL 0 mg
SODIUM 0 mg
POTASSIUM 385 mg
TOTAL CARBOHYDRATE 37 g
  DIETARY FIBER 3 g
  SUGARS 19 g
PROTEIN 2 g
PHOSPHORUS 40 mg

SUMMER FRUIT CLAFOUTI

SERVES: 6   **SERVING SIZE**: ¹/₆ recipe

Puffy on the outside, with a layer of melting berries underneath, this homestyle comfort food dessert has endless appeal. You can use peaches, plums, or any fruit in season for this recipe.

¹/₂ cup whole-wheat or unbleached white flour
¹/₄ cup quick-cooking rolled oats
¹/₂ teaspoon cinnamon
¹/₄ teaspoon salt
¹/₄ teaspoon nutmeg
 2 eggs, beaten
 6 ounces 2% or skim milk
 3 cups berries (or any combination of in-season fruit), halved or sliced
¹/₄ cup Splenda brown sugar blend
 1 teaspoon vanilla or almond extract
 1 teaspoon butter spread, such as Land O Lakes

1. Preheat oven to 375°F.

2. Make batter by mixing the flour, oats, and spices in a bowl. Gradually incorporate the liquid ingredients (eggs and milk) into the flour until a smooth mixture is formed.

3. Combine the fruit, Splenda brown sugar blend, and vanilla extract well in a small mixing bowl. Grease sides and bottom of a 1¹/₂-quart ceramic or glass baking dish with butter spread. Pour the mixture into the baking dish. Pour the batter over fruit.

4. Bake for approximately 25 minutes or until surface is puffy and golden brown.

5. Serve with plain or vanilla yogurt, sour cream, or whipped cream.

EXCHANGES
2 CARBOHYDRATE
¹/₂ FAT

CALORIES 160
  CALORIES FROM FAT 30
TOTAL FAT 3.5 g
  SATURATED FAT 1.2 g
  TRANS FAT 0.0 g
CHOLESTEROL 65 mg
SODIUM 140 mg
POTASSIUM 250 mg
TOTAL CARBOHYDRATE 28 g
  DIETARY FIBER 3 g
  SUGARS 13 g
PROTEIN 5 g
PHOSPHORUS 125 mg

INDEX

RECIPES

SUBJECT